Disclaimer: Please Read

The statements made in this guide have not been evaluated by the Food and Drug Administration and represent the professional opinion(s) of the author. The purpose of this book is not to act as a personal physician, coach, or healer to any reader and is not meant to directly or indirectly diagnose disease, dispense medical advice, or prescribe the use of any products or services as a treatment for sickness or disease. This information is for educational purposes only. You should always cooperate with a licensed health professional of your choice with the goal of creating optimal health. Please consult your physician prior to implementing any of the strategies mentioned in this book or starting any diet or exercise program—especially if you are pregnant or nursing. Any application or use of the information, resources, or recommendations contained in this book is at your own risk.

Copyright © 2018 Health Revival Partners

Author: Thomas J. Lewis, Ph.D.

ISBN: 9781790518753

Uncovering Chronic Inflammation & Hidden Infections

Thomas J. Lewis Ph.D.

Your immune system is constantly at war against invaders and stressors that lead to disease. Chronic disease develops when the immune system is weakened by any number of factors and is gradually overcome by inflammation, toxicity, and infectious burdens. We don't 'catch' diabetes or other chronic diseases, we slowly slip into a chronic disease state. What if you could accurately measure and identify immune attackers you have brewing right now? The Chronic Disease Temperature (CDT)™ biomarker panel does just that and provides you with the information you need to win the war and extend your health span.

HealthRevivalPartners.com

Uncovering Chronic Inflammation & Hidden Infections

Table of Contents

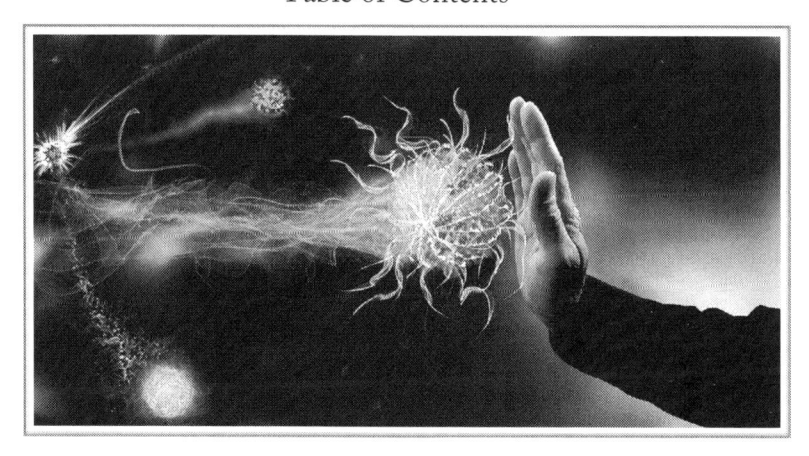

Chapter 1. Introduction

Chapter 2. What is My Immune System and How Does it Work?

Chapter 3. Why does My Immune System Backfire?

Chapter 4. Is My Immune System Weak or Strong?

Chapter 5. Markers of Immune Activity

Chapter 6. Measuring My Immune Activity

Chapter 7. Live Longer & Healthier

About the Author

References

Chapter 1. Introduction

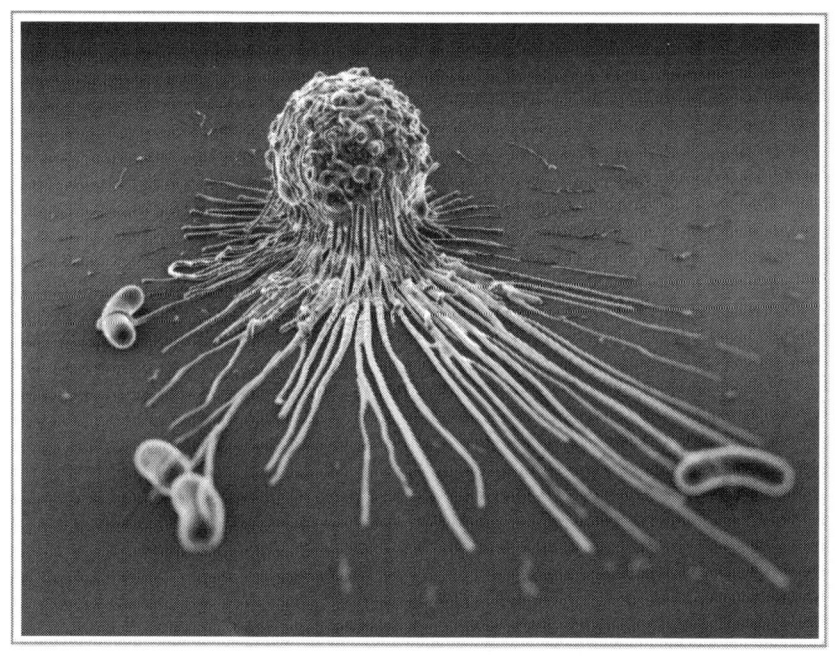

Your immune system is constantly at war against invaders and stressors that lead to disease. Chronic disease develops when the immune system is weakened by any number of factors and is gradually overcome by inflammation, toxicity, and infectious burdens. Along the path to chronic disease and poor health is a slow and often subtle change in your immune system that can be accurately measured. This is done by looking at immune cells and molecules themselves, and by measuring byproducts and disease-causing agents that engage your immune system. Measuring the strength of your immune system and its continued effort to keep you well will tell you where you are on the health-disease continuum.

1. Introduction

Our intent in this book is to help you recognize fact from fad as you work to improve your health. Take any approach that is right for you, but at the core, you need to accurately measure the impact of your efforts. Well-founded measurement is your armor against fads and incomplete science, enabling you to properly direct your personal health improvement efforts. In this book, I describe in detail, your immune system, how to measure it and suggest the next steps to improve its and your long-term health.

> *"If you are not testing you are guessing!"*

What is My Immune System?
Our immune system is the military defense complex of our body to fight disease-causing insults of any and all types. The military has many components - Army, Air Force, Navy, Marine, and Special Forces. So too does our immune system. It is comprised of the innate and adaptive systems. But it also contains other special defenses that support our primary security that we will refer to as "secondary" (2nd) and "tertiary" (3rd) components. The 2nd and 3rd parts of our immune system are working every day to keep us well and they especially kick into overdrive as we age and our primary immune system starts to deteriorate in a process called immunosenescence.

How does My Immune System Work?
Our immune system historically and primarily fights against infection and illness. It's a very intelligent system and can recognize the most subtle differences between the cells that make up our body and invaders and will try to get rid of anything unfamiliar. It may engulf a foreign substance, oxidize it with free

1. Introduction

radicals or place a bull's eye on it so another part of our immune system can seek and destroy it. It destroys germs (bacteria and viruses), parasites and grabs up foreign substances and objects bringing them to the right organs to filter, separate, break apart and remove.

Why does My Immune System Backfire?

On occasion, our defense system can cause collateral harm. Consider a virus and a piece of incompletely digested food. Both are strings of protein that are made from amino acid chains - the basic building blocks of life. The possible combination of amino acid chains are endless, yet our immune system keeps an accurate inventory of all these combinations that are fundamental to our specific makeup. When a foreign string of protein (bacteria, virus, parasite, prion, undigested food) gets into the bloodstream, our immune system may react or even overreact. This can also happen with seemingly harmless invaders such as pollen grains, causing an allergic reaction and autoimmune symptoms. But our immune system always has a reason for its action.

Is My Immune System Weak or Strong?

There is no specific laboratory test to determine the strength of your immune system but you inherently know how strong yours is compared to other people. If you are the one who withstands the flu or seldom gets colds, then you have a strong immune system. A favorite aunt of mine knew she was resilient because she always said "I'm not susceptible" when given the opportunity to avoid holding a child with a runny nose. Your immune system starts off, at the genesis of life, as a somewhat blank template partially influenced by genetics and epigenetics. After birth, however, you have the opportunity to 'mold the clay' of your immune health. The best way to measure your immune health is to assess the

1. Introduction

things that contribute to it - that being lifestyle, behaviors, and environment. Our Harvard Medical School and MIT team developed an immune health assessment survey that estimates your resistance toward chronic disease.

Markers of Immune Activity.

Our immune system is extraordinarily complex and elegant. However, regardless of the health problem, 'insult,' trauma or condition, 'usual suspects' are found to be working on our behalf keeping us healthy. These 'health protectors' range from white blood cells, to cytokines and other markers we view as inflammation. Understanding the connection between immune activation and inflammatory markers is important in understanding what your lab values mean and what you can do to reverse abnormal numbers and achieve better long-term health. Many of the most important markers of our chronic health show up in our blood and are easily and inexpensively measured.

Measuring My Immune Activity.

When your immune system is not being challenged and you feel well your immune system is relaxed - like troops hanging out in their quarters. Inflammation is an important measure of the activity of your immune system. Inflammation all too often gets a bad name but truly it is a sign that your immune system is fighting on your behalf. The question that needs to be answered is 'what is the inflammation fighting?'

Blood testing is the best way to measure inflammation and immune system activity. A strong immune system will react to a strong invader the same way a weak immune system will react to a weak invader. In both instances, it's easy to measure how piqued your immune system is. Common tests like white blood cell counts

1. Introduction

paint an accurate picture of inflammation and immune activity. The secret is in the interpretation of these tests. Most lab 'normal' values are looking at acute illness or if you already have a diagnosable disease. In this state, your immune system is on 'fire.' However, in essentially all cases of chronic disease, the markers of immune activity slowly elevate before reaching the 'fire' state. It's important to uncover a 'smoldering' immune system to be able to take proactive measures to protect your health.

Live Longer & Healthier.
Did you know that someone who lives to 100 enjoys 30 more years of better health compared to someone who lives to 80? Yes - that's 30 extra years of health-span. We often think of someone very old as decrepit. Sure they are when they are 99, but did you see them when they were 80? The secret to a long healthy life is measuring, understanding, and reversing risks. It's not about big risks. It is actually all about little risks adding up into a big problem. Consider a symphony where all the instruments and musicians play important roles. The same is true about health. We must ensure all parts of our health are working well together.

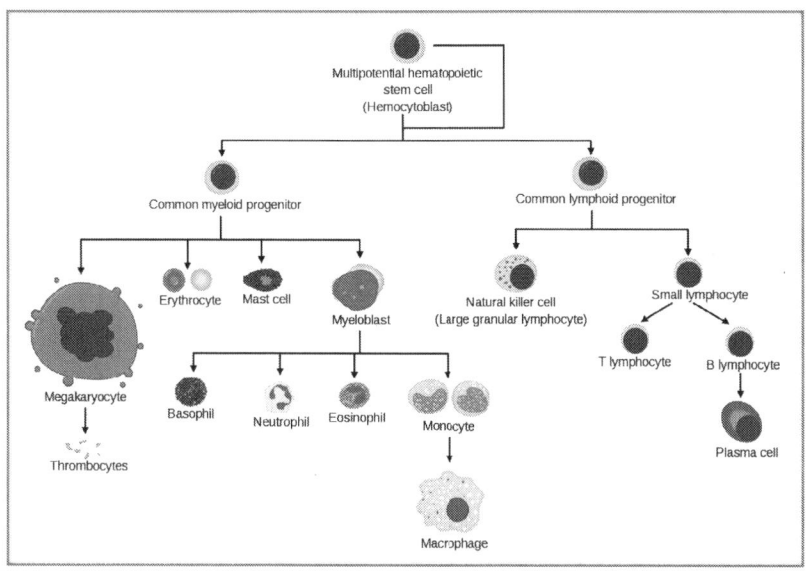

Chapter 2. What is My Immune System & How Does it Work?

Your immune system is your body's natural defense system. It's an intricate network of cells, tissues, and organs that band together to defend your body against invaders. Invaders such as bacteria, viruses, parasites, fungus, and toxins can all potentially make us sick. Most medical sources, from WebMD to the Mayo Clinic define our immune system as a defender against living, multiplying pathogens. [1] However, although most chronic diseases activate the immune system and it is so clear that it does so they are not explored or treated as diseases caused by pathogens!

> This is arguably the most interesting paradox
> in medicine today.

2. What is My Immune System & How Does it Work?

Pathogens and toxins can be found everywhere – in our homes, offices, water, air, and backyards. A healthy immune system protects us by first creating a barrier that stops those invaders (antigens) from entering our body. If one slips by the barrier, the immune system produces white blood cells, and other substances and proteins that attack and destroy these foreign substances, that is according to its ability and based on immune system strength. Your immune system seeks to find the antigen and get rid of it before it can reproduce (as is the case with pathogens) or collect (as is the case with toxins). In the next phase, the immune system revs up, even more, to destroy the invaders as they multiply.

The immune system adapts, over time, to recognize millions of different antigens. That's why it's important to get exposure to our natural environment.

"The Dose Makes the Poison"

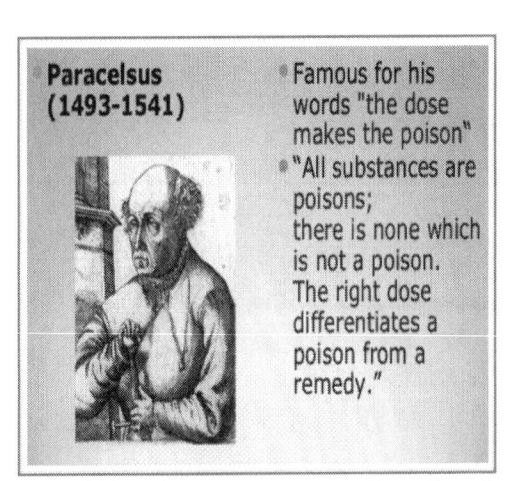

Paracelsus (1493-1541)
- Famous for his words "the dose makes the poison"
- "All substances are poisons; there is none which is not a poison. The right dose differentiates a poison from a remedy."

This is true in both Chemistry and Medicine. Simply put, a small amount of a bad thing may not be harmful, and sometimes may actually be beneficial. On the other hand, too much of a good thing may be dangerous. Consider too much oxygen that is essential to life yet will lead to harm and even death if taken in excess. Our immune system protects us from exposure by developing a tolerance to an insult or attempting to eradicate it completely. This is the basic definition of immunity. Our immune

2. What is My Immune System & How Does it Work?

system can produce what it needs to eliminate nearly everything if we arm it with the right resources.

Our immune system, like a muscle, grows stronger when it is challenged - for example - by fighting against some stressor. Lifting a heavy weight is a stressor (insult), so is an exposure to a virus. When our military troops are out on maneuvers practicing for the big battle, they are developing a strong immunity against the enemy. You need to train your immune system to be ready to save your life or protect you from a stealth (hidden) invader trying to take you down from within. Lyme disease is a classic example of a stealth, and often very patient, invader.

When it's well equipped, this elaborate immune defense system can keep health problems at bay, ranging from cancer to the common cold. We now know, based on the 2018 Nobel Prize in Medicine, that cancer can evade the immune system.[2] It does so by shutting down the production of certain immune cells that would normally sense and destroy the cancer cells. However, this happens only when you have diagnosable, or at least, advancing cancer. All of us have some cancer in our bodies and our defense is constantly detecting, destroying, and removing these cells so we remain 'cancer free.'[3] Again, the dose makes the poison.

If your immune system is weak, the insult that drives the proliferation of cancer multiply with ease. When these cells or substances reach a high enough "dose" it (the virus, toxin, or cancer) effectively turns down your immune system and the cancer is able to grow uncontrolled. The recent Nobel Prize in Medicine research confirms that there are profound and manageable solutions to cancer. Specifically, know the strength of your immune system and work to enhance it every day. By doing so the

2. What is My Immune System & How Does it Work?

cancer cells are much less likely to reach the dose necessary to grow uncontrolled.

The true miracle of immunity is an elaborate and dynamic communications network. Millions of cells, organized into sets and subsets, gather like clouds of bees swarming around a hive and pass information back and forth. Once immune cells receive the alarm, they undergo tactical changes and begin to produce powerful substances like peroxide that oxidize and destroy membranes of evaders, killing them. Some of these substances allow the cells to regulate their own growth and behavior, enlist their fellows, and direct new recruits to trouble spots.

Innate Immune System: The innate immune system is made of defenses against infection that can be activated immediately once a pathogen attacks. The innate immune system is essentially made up of barriers that aim to keep viruses, bacteria, parasites, and other foreign particles out of your body or limit their ability to spread and move throughout the body. The innate immune system includes:

- Physical Barriers - such as skin, the gastrointestinal tract, the respiratory tract, the nasopharynx, cilia, eyelashes, and other body hair.

- Defense Mechanisms - such as secretions, mucus, bile, gastric acid, saliva, tears, and sweat.

- General Immune Responses - such as immune cells, inflammation, complement, and non-specific cellular responses. The inflammatory response actively brings immune cells to the site of an infection by increasing blood flow to the area. Complement is an immune response that marks pathogens for destruction and makes holes in the cell

2. What is My Immune System & How Does it Work?

membrane of the pathogen.

The innate immune system is always general, or nonspecific, meaning anything that it identified as foreign or non-self is a target for the innate immune response. The innate immune system is activated by the presence of antigens and their chemical properties.

White blood cells (leukocytes) work to defend and protect the human body as part of the innate immune system. In order to patrol the entire body, leukocytes travel by way of the circulatory system. Their primary modes of action are to engulf and consume or to kill the invading pathogen with a toxin, generally an oxidizing agent like peroxide. Each of the various white blood cells has a special role within the immune system. Many are able to transform themselves in different ways.

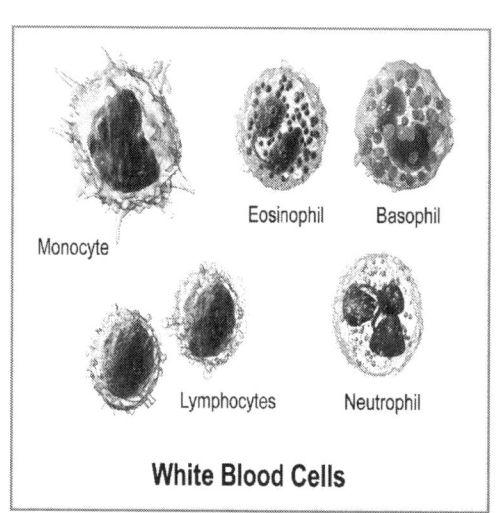

Many of these cells are easily measured with a simple blood test. Their levels tell a lot about the health of your immune system, the extent to which your system is under attack and how well you are doing in your war against chronic disease.

Neutrophils, the most common white blood cells, have a short lifespan - generally less than a day. Once in the blood neutrophils can move through capillary walls into tissue. They are attracted to

2. What is My Immune System & How Does it Work?

foreign material, particularly bacteria. If you get a splinter or a cut, neutrophils are attracted. Once a neutrophil finds a foreign particle or a bacterium, the neutrophils engulf it, releasing enzymes, hydrogen peroxide and other chemicals to kill it. When there is a serious infection, pus will form. Pus is just dead neutrophils and other debris from the battlefield.

Eosinophils and basophils are less common than neutrophils. Eosinophils focus on parasites in the skin and the lungs. Basophils carry histamine and are important for causing inflammation. For the immune system, inflammation is good. It brings in more blood and dilates capillary walls so more immune system cells can get to the infection. This is why stimulating inflammation is an emerging strategy for treating specific inflammatory conditions and why added plasma rich in immune molecules is beneficial to recovery. [4] [5]

Monocytes are the biggest of all blood cells. Monocytes are released by bone marrow, float in the bloodstream, enter tissue and become macrophages. Most boundary tissue has its own macrophages. For example, alveolar macrophages keep the lungs clean by ingesting foreign particles like dust and smoke. One of their jobs is to remove dead neutrophils (or pus) as part of the healing process.

The lymphocytes handle most bacterial and viral infections. Lymphocytes start in bone marrow. Those that will become B cells develop in the bone marrow before entering the blood. T cells start in the bone marrow but migrate through the bloodstream to the thymus, where they mature. T cells and B cells tend to concentrate in lymph tissue including the lymph nodes, the thymus, and the spleen. Lymphopenia (low lymphocytes) is frequent in advanced cancers and predicts the toxicity of chemotherapy. [6] It can also

2. What is My Immune System & How Does it Work?

occur in response to infection, severe stress, chronic disease, or malnutrition.

T cells actually bump up against cells and kill them. One type of T cell known as a killer T cell can detect cells in the body that are harboring viruses. When it detects such a cell it kills it. Other T cells, called Helper and Suppressor T cells, help make killer T cells and control the immune response.

Another innate response type of lymphocyte, known as a natural killer or NK cell, comes from the same place as T cells. NK cells respond quickly to several kinds of foreign substances and are specialized in killing cancer cells and virus-infected cells.

Adaptive (Acquired) Immune System: Colds don't last forever, the flu isn't as bad the 3rd time, and you don't seem as susceptible to your grandchild's sniffles as you were towards that of your own child. Unlike the innate immune system, which attacks based on the identification of general threats, the adaptive immunity is activated by exposure to pathogens and other insults and uses an immunological memory to learn about the threat and enhance the immune response accordingly. A person who recovers from measles, for example, is protected for life against measles by the adaptive immune system, although not against other common viruses such as those that cause mumps or chickenpox.

Any substance capable of eliciting an adaptive immune response is referred to as an antigen. Remarkably, the adaptive immune system can distinguish between antigens that are very similar -such as between two proteins that differ in only a single amino acid. [7] The adaptive immune response is much slower to respond to threats and infections, at least the first time it responds to a new antigen,

2. What is My Immune System & How Does it Work?

compared to the innate immune response, which is primed and ready to fight at all times.

Adaptive immune responses are carried out by lymphocytes. There are two broad classes of such responses, cell-mediated immune responses and antibody responses, each carried out by different classes of lymphocytes, the T and B cells. Both B cells and T cells are lymphocytes that are derived from specific types of stem cells, called multipotent hematopoietic stem cells, in the bone marrow. After they are made in the bone marrow, they need to mature and become activated. Each type of cell follows different paths to their final, mature forms.

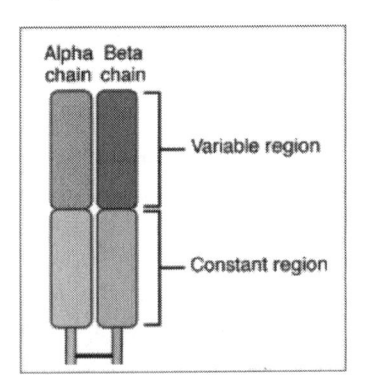

The T lymphocytes are particularly important, as they not only control a multitude of immune responses directly but also control B cell immune responses in many cases as well. Thus, many of the decisions about how to attack a pathogen are made at the T cell level.

T lymphocytes recognize antigens based on a two-chain protein including a variable region affording almost infinite specificity (see image left).

In antibody responses, B cells are activated to secrete antibodies, which are proteins called immunoglobulins. The antibodies circulate in the bloodstream and permeate the other body fluids, where they bind specifically to the

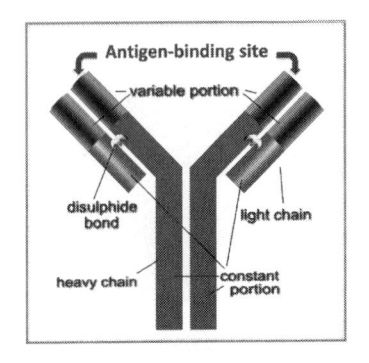

2. What is My Immune System & How Does it Work?

foreign antigen that stimulated their production at the "variable region."

When a pathogen is present or tries to return, the B cell clones itself to produce millions of antibodies designed to eliminate the germ. Binding of antibody, in the "variable portion" of the antibody shown in the diagram, inactivates viruses and microbial toxins by blocking their ability to bind to receptors on our own cells. Antibody binding also marks invading pathogens for destruction, mainly by making it easier for phagocytic cells of the innate immune system to ingest them.

Tertiary Immunity: This third layer of immunity runs alongside our innate and adaptive immune system. It is always present and keeps us healthy later in life when our immune system slowly declines (immunosenescence), yet few people understand what it really is. In order to understand this part of your immune system, you must accept a very simple but highly controversial concept.

> Your body ONLY produces substances that help you either thrive or survive.

2. What is My Immune System & How Does it Work?

<u>Cholesterol:</u> This most vilified of all substances the body produces

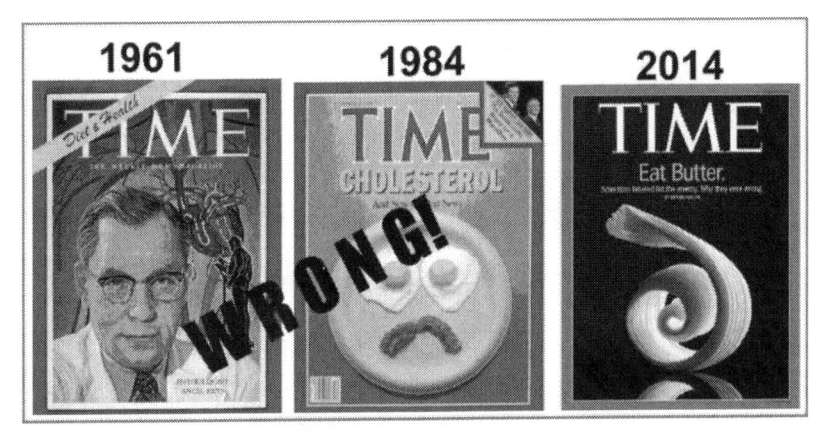

is actually one of the most important. [8] [9] [10]

- Cholesterol plays a role in forming and maintaining cell membranes and structures.
- Cholesterol can insert between fat molecules making up the cell, making the membrane more fluid. Cells also need cholesterol to help them adjust to changes in temperature.
- Cholesterol is essential for making a number of critical hormones, including the stress hormone cortisol. Cholesterol is also used to make sex hormones testosterone, progesterone, and estrogen.
- The liver also uses cholesterol to make bile, a fluid that plays a vital role in the processing and digestion of fats.
- Cholesterol is used by nerve cells for insulation.
- Your body also needs cholesterol to make vitamin D. In the presence of sunlight, cholesterol is converted into vitamin D.
- Cholesterol has antibiotic properties and high levels of cholesterol were shown to reduce mortality in AIDS patients. [11]
- Cholesterol is a natural antibiotic. [12]

Cholesterol, seeking its appropriate level as governed by our body, is an extremely important part of our immune response. [13, 14, 15] New

2. What is My Immune System & How Does it Work?

research is showing if your cholesterol is too low, the chance of getting cancer or dying from a violent death like suicide increases. [16] Cholesterol is a building block for cells and membranes. Twenty-five percent (25%) of the cholesterol in our body is in our brain and our brain is only 2.5% the mass of our body. Therefore, 10 times more cholesterol is in our brain compared to other body tissue. It's there for a reason.

In older people, it is now known that having a blood cholesterol greater than 240 mg/dL lowers risk of sudden death and increases life expectancy. [17] High cholesterol levels are positively correlated with longevity, especially in the elderly, most likely by helping curb infection. A paper titled, "Total cholesterol and risk of mortality in the oldest old" affirms this statement. [18] Let's put this data into manageable terms for those of you focused on a long and healthy life, in other words, becoming the oldest of the old. The table below shows favorable life and health span with increasing cholesterol levels - as we age.

Total cholesterol mg/dL	Mortality Rate per 100 person-years	Relative Risk of Death
<160	11	1.52: 52% *increase*
161-199	7	1.00
200-240	5	0.77: 23% decrease
>240	4	0.69: 39% decrease

Mortality rates GO DOWN as cholesterol levels GO UP.

Indeed very high cholesterol (>300) in midlife is cause for alarm, but the cholesterol is not to blame. Those with high cholesterol before they are elderly are ill and need to be properly diagnosed and treated. Then their cholesterol will come down to levels appropriate for their physiology. Older people have inflammation –

2. What is My Immune System & How Does it Work?

it is just a fact of life and aging. Elevated cholesterol is there to protect you against some of the inevitable ravages of aging.

Cholesterol is a marker that should not be ignored. Elevated cholesterol is a sign of excess inflammation or infection and that your innate and adaptive immune systems are in need of assistance, regardless of age. Find the cause of elevated cholesterol and, to protect your long-term health, don't lower it artificially.

<u>Amyloid Formations:</u> These formations, like cholesterol, are considered toxic in our bodies. Amyloidosis is considered a disease of abnormal proteins - proteins formed in a 'so-called' misfolded conformation. But are they really abnormal or an appropriate response from an active immune system? WebMD calls amyloidosis "a serious health problem that can lead to life-threatening organ failure." Sources like Mayo Clinic claim, "Amyloidosis is a rare disease that occurs when a substance called amyloid builds up in your organs." Are they right or just professing the current dogma?

Beta-amyloid, a type of amyloid formation, is the main "villain" of Alzheimer's disease. After hundreds of clinical trials that successfully reduced the level of beta-amyloid, and nearly $1 trillion dollars spent, not one study participant with Alzheimer's showed any improvement. [19] These Alzheimer's amyloid plaques may actually be part of the immune system, a new study has revealed. The research carried out at Harvard Medical School indicates that amyloid-beta may be the 'first line of defense' against infection in the brain and other tissues. [20] [21] The Harvard team reports, "Members of this evolutionarily ancient family of proteins, collectively known as antimicrobial peptides (AMPs), share many of the amyloid's purportedly abnormal activities." [22]

2. What is My Immune System & How Does it Work?

Research Translation: Amyloids are a natural response by our immune system against infection.

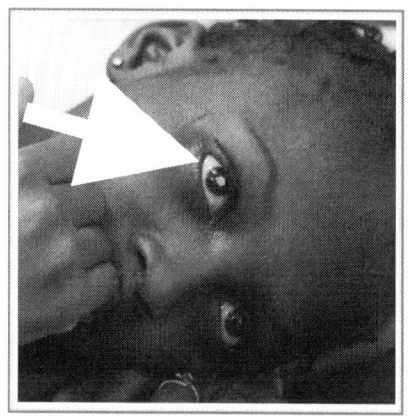

Individuals with severe, chronic inflammatory conditions lasting several years deposit amyloid in many tissues and this is a fairly common condition despite prevailing doctrine. Cataract, a very common eye condition, and the #1 surgery performed throughout the world is an example of amyloid formation.

In this image, note the white formation in the center of the eye of this 5-year-old child. She was infected with Ebola and survived. A natural response to the disease was an amyloid formation that is commonly called a cataract. Research from Harvard Medical School dating back to 2003 shows that cataracts are a type of amyloid and they actually form to protect us from infection. [23, 24] It's highly likely that this child has amyloid formations throughout her body.

All this new information indicate that amyloid and other substances not well understood but produced by our body mount a natural protective response to disease and by responding to infection. [25]

The common thread between all the immune cells of the innate, adaptive and tertiary immune system is that they primarily defend against infection. Could it be that modern medicine is looking at the wrong disease-causing culprits and we have to look back at history when infectious disease was the major recognized cause of disease?

2. What is My Immune System & How Does it Work?

"The textbooks say, in 1900 most people died of infectious diseases, and today most people don't die of infectious disease; they die of cancer and heart disease and Alzheimer's and all these things. Well, in time I think the textbooks will have to be rewritten to say, 'Throughout history, most people have died of infectious disease, and most people continue to die of infectious disease.'" [1]

- Dr. Paul Ewald - Evolutionary Biologist

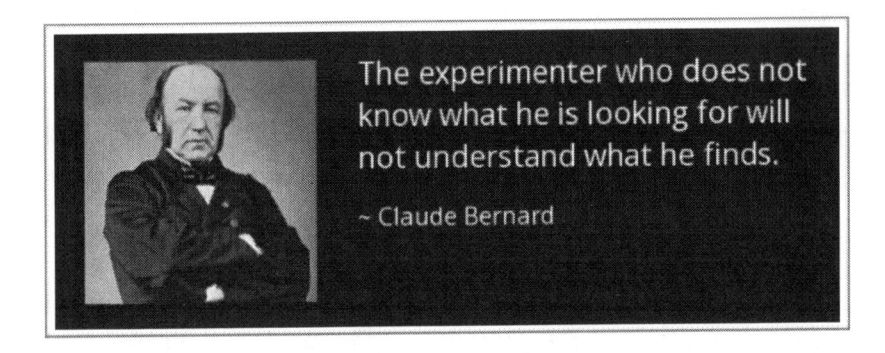

> The experimenter who does not know what he is looking for will not understand what he finds.
>
> ~ Claude Bernard

Chapter 3. Why does My Immune System Backfire?

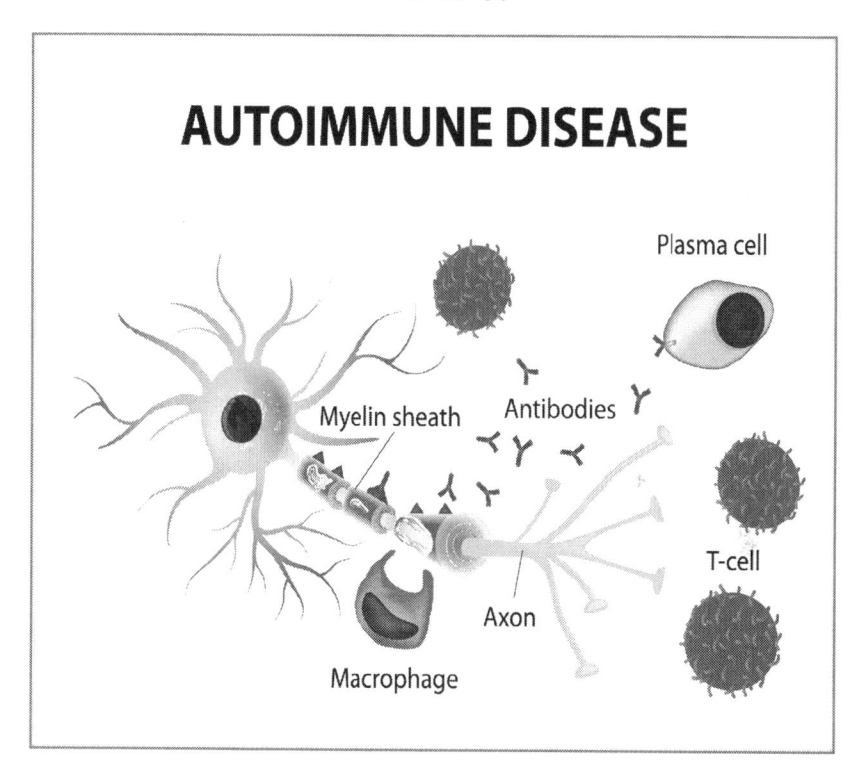

AUTOIMMUNE DISEASE

- Plasma cell
- Myelin sheath
- Antibodies
- T-cell
- Axon
- Macrophage

In most cases, when our body appears to attack itself for no reason, it's doing exactly what WE programmed it to do. Our body never deliberately backfires to harm us - rather it is always trying to protect us from a perceived threat. However, there can be collateral damage when a clever organism or another protein or toxin that shouldn't be in our body looks like a part of our body. This concept is called "molecular mimicry" which is defined as: "the theoretical possibility that sequence similarities between foreign and self-peptides are sufficient to result in the cross-activation of our adaptive immune system." [26]

3. Why does My Immune System Backfire?

There are many different views on autoimmunity, most of which are opinions based on observation - rather than from a rigorous scientific investigation. Consider the following examples that align with our philosophy that your immune system is nearly perfect, especially when it is given the supplies it needs to function at peak efficiency. It's our lack of understanding of its action that leads us to believe that it backfires.

Example 1: Carolyn is a healthy 12-year-old with a severe nut allergy. Her family brought Carolyn to a nutritionist who enrolled her in a program called Allergy Release Technique. After 1 year of immune system training, she overcame her nut allergy completely. [27] According to the nutritionist, "a special computer program helps identify stressors in the body. I also use something similar to acupressure to help strengthen my patients' immune systems. All of the kids I treat also take a high-quality probiotic." The issue with Carolyn was a lack of exposure to natural substances early in life, during her initial immune system development, thus something as natural as a nut appeared to be an antigen (foreign).

Example 2: Toxic chemicals can impact the body in the same way as a harmful or unrecognized substance in food. There are chemicals known as "sensitizers." A sensitizer is defined by OSHA as "a chemical that causes a substantial proportion of exposed people or animals to develop an allergic reaction in normal tissue after repeated exposure to the chemical." The condition of being sensitized to a chemical is called chemical hypersensitivity. The most common symptoms are skin rashes and respiratory issues like wheezing. This sounds similar to Celiac and autoimmunity, doesn't it?

Chemical sensitivity does not always happen upon a first exposure - it frequently does so after a long history of repeated exposures.

3. Why does My Immune System Backfire?

This process has many parallels to type 2 diabetes and lung cancer induced by smoking, among other chronic diseases. There is a long period of tolerance followed by a dramatic response by the body to the daily, continual insult. In the case of the allergy or chemical sensitivity, it really appears that the immune system is sending us a signal that we are getting to the point of no return and it's time to stop harming ourselves. With food, the message is to stop taking in that toxic, irritating, or unrecognized food.

Why do some people develop sensitivities while others do not? The truth most likely lies somewhere in our history. The NY Times in an article titled, "Feed Your Kids Peanuts, Early and Often, New Guidelines Urge," explains that early exposure conditions the body to develop the necessary means to properly deal with the digestion of harmful parts of any food. [28] Alternatively, when exposed early in life, your body simply recognizes something that shouldn't be harmful as just that - not harmful.

Stealth infection is often an under-diagnosed contributor to autoimmune symptoms. In a paper titled, "The role of Infections in Autoimmune Diseases," the authors state: "There are more than 80 identified autoimmune diseases. [29] Multiple factors are thought to contribute to the development of immune response to self, including genetics, age, and environment." In particular, viruses, bacteria, and other infectious pathogens are the major postulated environmental triggers of autoimmunity. [30] In cases of infection, it's not really autoimmunity, but rather a response by our immune system to quell an otherwise undetected chronic infection. Maybe there is a lot less true autoimmunity than we originally thought? The key to answering this question is more thorough diagnostics.

3. Why does My Immune System Backfire?

We know all drugs have side effects and they are not natural substances so our immune system will often react to them, creating additional stress in our bodies. Many drugs impact the health of our gut, contributing to autoimmune diseases. Extensive new research shows that people on stomach acid reducing drugs have much less healthy gut microbiomes. These people have more frequent cases of infections and autoimmune disorders. [31] [32] There continues to be a very rapid rise in gut and autoimmune diseases in the U.S. and developing countries that have adopted a 'westernization' of lifestyle.

Acid neutralizing drugs are not the only ones that can disrupt the gut-to-blood vessel barrier normally maintained by our adaptive and innate immunity. Several important recent studies have suggested an association between oral contraceptive, menopausal hormone therapy and the risk for these diseases. [33] PPIs, a type of antacid and contraceptives, may reduce absorption of important nutrients and induce inflammation, contributing to gut dysbiosis and autoimmune conditions.

According to and article titled, *Gut microbes are vulnerable to wide range of drugs* "Anti-inflammatories, antipsychotics and cancer drugs are among a host of medications that might inadvertently slow the growth of gut bacteria. Many antibiotics can upset digestion, but it has not been clear to what extent other types of drug affect the gut's bacterial balance. Athanasios Typas at the European Molecular Biology Laboratory in Heidelberg, Germany, and his colleagues tested the effect of 835 non-antibiotic drugs on 40 common gut bacteria. Roughly one-quarter of the drugs restrained the growth of at least one bacterium, and nearly 5% affected at least ten. The authors also found that patients taking these non-antibiotics often have side effects similar to those reported for antibiotics." [34]

3. Why does My Immune System Backfire?

Mood disorders and even Alzheimer's are now considered part of the autoimmune spectrum. Gastrointestinal inflammation tied to an inadequate gut microbiome is strongly associated with a proliferation of infection and disease. The inflammation triggers 'autoimmunity' in a couple of ways. First, the inflammation leads to gut permeability with harmful substances easily getting into the bloodstream. Second, antagonistic pathogens are able to multiply when beneficial bacteria are compromised. Third, the change in the gut environment creates a vicious cycle allowing this downward spiral of more inflammation, permeability, and infection to continue.

The emerging field of microbiome research lies at the center of these interactions with evidence that the abundance and diversity of resident gut microbiota contribute to digestion, inflammation, gut permeability, health, and disease. [35] Lagging behind in research and implementation in society is the importance of early-in-life exposure to microbes that populate our gut beneficially.

Did you ever wonder why a toddler puts things in their mouth? Even though the concept of chewing on grass or swallowing a little dirt seems repulsive, can we agree that it's more natural compared to sucking on a plastic toy make "who knows where?"

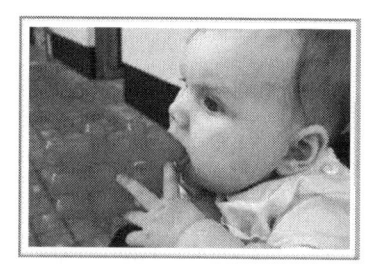

Versus

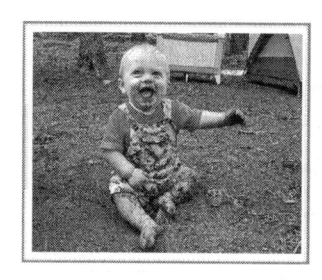

3. Why does My Immune System Backfire?

The challenge an autoimmune sufferer faces is a lack of appreciation of causation by many conventional doctors. This is due, in part, to the cryptic nature of infection. That is, a person may have been infected years or even decades before a symptom erupts thus the connection between disease and the infecting agent is not made. The organism(s) of Lyme disease is a prime example. Someone may have bitten by a tick in their youth yet did not develop disease until later in life when their immune system was compromised.

Another, perhaps more important issue, is that of lab value interpretation. Most conventional doctors are looking for the 'fire' of disease in biomarkers. They are only looking for 'acute' disease and answering the question, "are you going to get very sick, have a heart attack, or die today?'

While most chronic diseases appear to come on suddenly, they actually creek up slowly. The issue is lab normal values in the standard-of-care are really not normal. They don't have the predictive power to measure changes on the way to a serious disease condition. Medicine is not looking for "smoldering" disease.

Further, the only marker being watched closely is cholesterol. Its normal value several decades ago was 270mg/dL, then it was dropped to 240, and now it is 200. Today more than 75% of people who have a first heart attack don't even have elevated cholesterol levels by these most recent standards. [36] Is the level of normal still too high or are we looking at an inappropriate cause of disease?

Many immune markers do paint a very vivid picture of smoldering inflammation and chronic disease susceptibility. White blood cell

3. Why does My Immune System Backfire?

counts and markers of inflammation like c-reactive protein and homocysteine, when only slightly elevated, thus 'normal' yet well within normal limits, tell a story about stealth infection, sensitivities, and inflammation that should not be ignored. These markers provide an early warning sign for chronic disease in general and often provide a clue as to the cause of our immune system backfiring or over-reacting. In the final analysis, our immune system is doing exactly what we trained it to do and is supposed to do - protect us.

4. Is My Immune System Weak or Strong?

Chapter 4. Is My Immune System Weak or Strong?

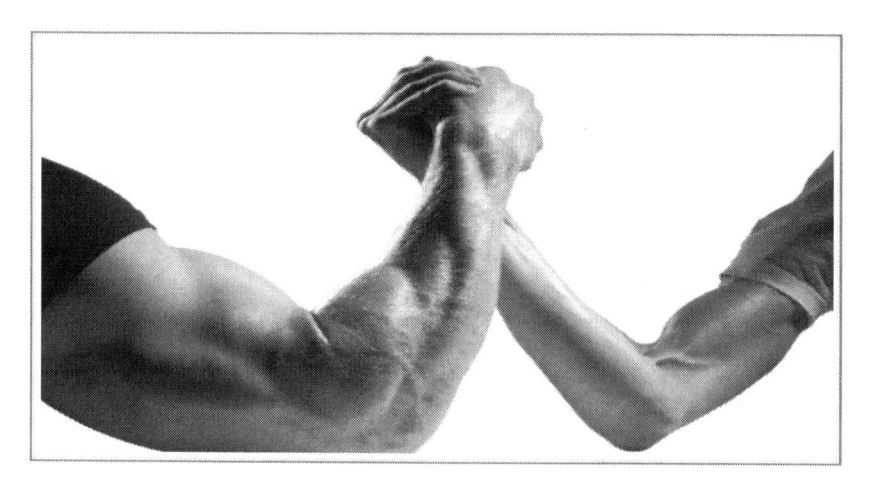

Knowing the strength of your immune health and why it is either weak or strong is the first critical step towards its optimization.

How your immune system responds to stresses and challenges is easily measured by performing laboratory tests for inflammation and actual immune cell activity. Measuring the strength of your immune system, objectively, presents a challenge because so many factors may influence the magnitude of the response. However, through a little self-evaluation, we can all intuitively gage our own immune system health. For example, do you catch that cold circulating in the office? Do you recover quickly from an injury? Are you pain-free or suffering from chronic pain? The answers to these questions tell us a lot about your immune health status.

Attempts continue to be made to measure immune health. For example, in a study of 24 people, the authors of, "Measuring the

4. Is My Immune System Weak or Strong?

immune system: a comprehensive approach for the analysis of immune functions in humans," indicate that immune health is a combination of many extrinsic and intrinsic factors such as exposure to chemicals, stress, nutrition, and age. [37] They demonstrated the feasibility to detect changes in immune functions. However, they did not measure comparative immune health.

Our immune systems vary as a consequence of heritable and non-heritable influences, but symbiotic and pathogenic microbes and other non-heritable influences, such as environment and lifestyle, explain most of this variation. Understanding when and how such influences shape the human immune system is key to defining health and understanding the risk of inflammatory and infectious diseases. [38]

The best way, we have concluded, to estimate your relative immune system strength & health is to compare (1) health risk factors like lifestyle, behavior, and environment to (2) immune system blood biomarkers. When these two measurements align, then your immune strength is revealed by the health risk factors. Importantly you have control over risk factors - thus you have control over your own immune system strength.

You have substantial control over your immune system strength.

Measuring immune strength by measuring sickness and disease susceptibility is not a new concept. Functional medicine is particularly good at this type of assessment. The Institute for Functional Medicine members developed and uses a

4. Is My Immune System Weak or Strong?

comprehensive intake form to determine your health status. Within that form are dozens of questions to assess your life and health risk. What is lacking is the intelligence of the intake form to develop an individualized risk profile based on your unique set of risks.

We have developed a sophisticated algorithm to measure your immune health status, referred to as your Chronic Disease Assessment (CDA)™. It is a comprehensive health risk assessment tool developed by a team of doctors and scientists from Harvard Medical School and MIT. This patent-pending technology evolved from patient-centered clinical work through iterative evaluation of patient risks, their medical and personal history, and clinical outcomes. In addition, the current CDA incorporates analytics developed by hundreds of doctors of functional medicine. It is a complete series of questions, derived from best-of-breed functional intake forms, known health risk factors, and our own clinical experience.

The responses to this survey have been compared to a statistically valid number of corresponding immune health blood labs, which is discussed in detail in the next chapter. Artificial intelligence was applied to ensure a strong statistical correlation between data obtained and biomarker values. The result is a straightforward, yet elegant linear correlation between life risks and biomarkers. [39]

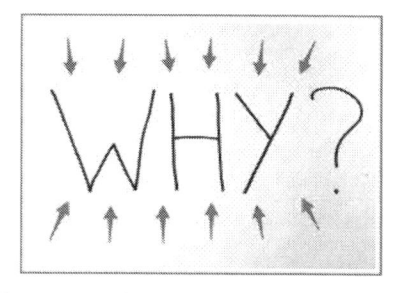

The life risk score is a measure of your current immune system health. A free mini version of the CDA is, called "Your Risk at a Glance," is available as a sample of our more robust screening tool,

4. Is My Immune System Weak or Strong?

to take on our website.

The comprehensive CDA answers the Question "WHY." Why am I at risk or do I have chronic health problems? Further, it addresses three very important questions about health and risk:

1. What is your susceptibility for future disease?
2. What is your prognosis for recovery, debilitation, or survival if you have a diagnosis like cancer, diabetes, heart disease or Alzheimer's?
3. What are your areas of highest risk?

The CDA generates a detailed risk report, and one of our coaches will work closely with you, providing practical solutions available to address every identified risk.

The proven fundamental concept of the CDA is that poor health is a collection of many small risks. This approach is empowering to individuals, even those in a high-risk category because single risks are relatively easy to eliminate. This concept liberates you, the individual, to take control over your quality of life and health span. It is common knowledge that eating fast food daily, not exercising, and smoking creates health risks that often lead to disease. But, there are many other risks that increase a person's chance of disease or a poor prognosis that are neglected yet offer a real opportunity to improve your overall health status.

For instance, in 2010 the French smoked at twice the rate of Americans, 28% of the adult population compared to 14%. According to well-documented statistics and the "French Paradox," the French have 1/3rd the heart disease morbidity and mortality. A clever biostatistician might conclude that "smoking

4. Is My Immune System Weak or Strong?

reduces the likelihood of dying from heart disease by 600%!" The proper conclusion is that the average French person has many fewer chronic life risks compared to Americans.

Correlating life risks with biomarkers is an emerging activity in the new P4 medicine (Predictive, Preventive, Personalized and Participatory) and is gaining interest. [40]

The CDA, being a series of questions, is a subjective measure of life risk. Biometrics are objective thus provide a more realistic risk score. In this instance, however, the CDA was developed as a companion to a novel biometric panel - the Chronic Disease Temperature (CDT)™, discussed in depth in the next chapter. The chart on the following page is the correlation between the CDA and CDT. The strong correlation between the two measures gives great confidence in the power of the life risk assessment to determine actual health risk - and immune strength. In addition, the risk assessment provides insights into solutions to improve health while a biomarker panel does not. Reverse as many of those little risks as you can!

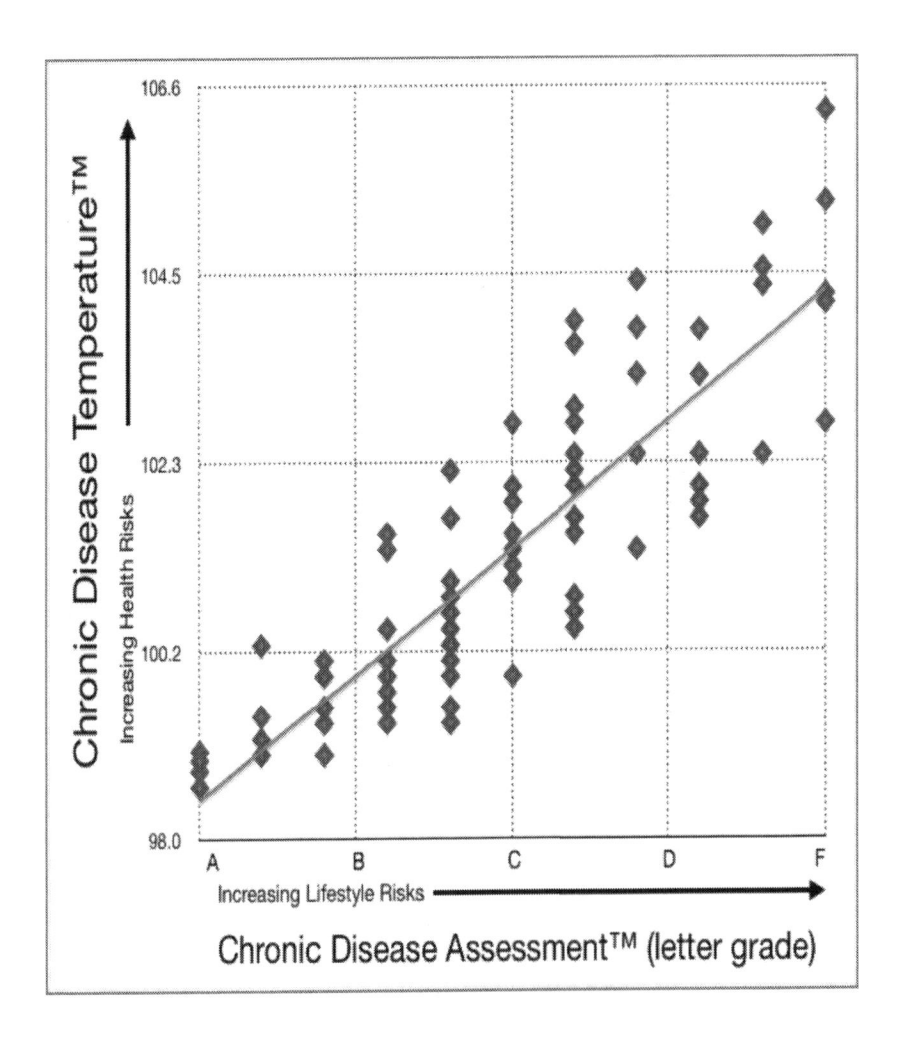

5. Markers of Immune Activity

Chapter 5. Markers of Immune Activity

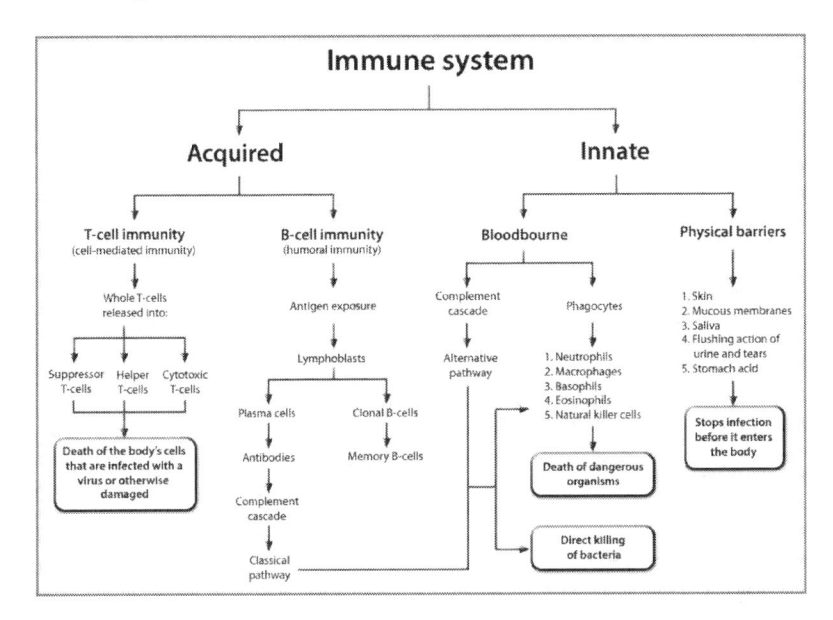

```
                            Immune system
                                 |
                ┌────────────────┴────────────────┐
             Acquired                           Innate
                │                                 │
       ┌────────┴────────┐              ┌─────────┼──────────┐
  T-cell immunity   B-cell immunity   Bloodbourne      Physical barriers
 (cell-mediated      (humoral                              │
   immunity)         immunity)                      1. Skin
        │                │                          2. Mucous membranes
   Whole T-cells    Antigen exposure                3. Saliva
   released into:        │                          4. Flushing action of
                    Lymphoblasts                       urine and tears
                                                    5. Stomach acid
```

(Acquired → T-cell: Suppressor T-cells, Helper T-cells, Cytotoxic T-cells → Death of the body's cells that are infected with a virus or otherwise damaged)

(B-cell: Lymphoblasts → Plasma cells, Clonal B-cells; Plasma cells → Antibodies; Clonal B-cells → Memory B-cells; Antibodies → Complement cascade → Classical pathway)

(Bloodbourne: Complement cascade → Alternative pathway; Phagocytes: 1. Neutrophils, 2. Macrophages, 3. Basophils, 4. Eosinophils, 5. Natural killer cells → Death of dangerous organisms; Classical/Alternative pathway → Direct killing of bacteria)

(Physical barriers → Stops infection before it enters the body)

The immune system is both elegant and complex. Fortunately, several 'usual suspects' show up in our peripheral blood that let us know our immune system is engaged in the battle of life. The blood biomarkers included in this chapter allow us to measure your immune activity precisely and accurately.

There are many types of tests including saliva; stool, urine, imaging, and blood, but our experience suggests the markers in the blood best reflect what is going on in your body both acutely and chronically. Blood biomarkers change by either elevating or lowering in response to insult. When these markers stay in an abnormal range, even just slightly, for extended periods of time, chronic disease and poor health may develop.

Cytokines

Cytokines are the scouts of any war party. These cells are constantly sending out signals to let other cells know what's going

5. Markers of Immune Activity

on. Cytokines that are a group of proteins secreted by cells of the immune system, act as chemical messengers. Cytokines released from one cell affect the actions of other cells by binding to receptors on their surface. You can think of these receptors as your phone. They receive the cytokine's chemical "text" message, and

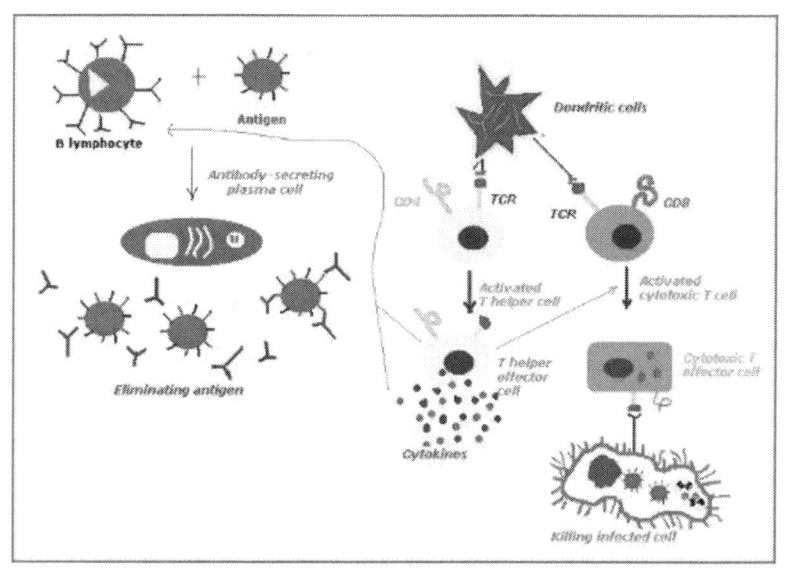

then the receiving cell performs activities based on that message. There are different types of cytokines, including chemokines, interferons, interleukins, lymphokines, and tumor necrosis factor. They can act alone, work together or maybe even work against each other, but ultimately the role of cytokines is to help regulate the immune response. Cytokines are involved in many aspects of inflammation and immunity. In fact, you can thank the different cytokines for triggering some familiar symptoms that arise when your body fights an infection, such as fever, inflammation, and pain. Also, these cytokines may be only slightly elevated when fighting a low-grade chronic infection or disease. Their levels in our body tell us a great deal about our current state, and more importantly, our future state of health.

5. Markers of Immune Activity

Cytokines complement the innate immune system and are produced following infection. They are active in stimulating phagocytic cells, monocytes, macrophages, neutrophils, and endothelial cells to react against, or bind to, micro-organisms, and to summon other immune cells to the site of infection. There has been a recent explosion of information on cytokines, their complex interactions, and maturation that lead to effective immune responses. [41]

Interferons are proteins that inhibit viruses from replicating. If a cell gets invaded by a virus, it releases interferons. This signals other cells to put up their shields so the virus does not spread. So Interferons interfere with the spread of a virus. Interferons also activate natural killer T-Cells. These cells extend the fight against the virus by destroying infected cells.

Interleukins are cytokine proteins that regulate immune and inflammatory responses. They are an essential part for the functioning of both the innate and adaptive systems. Interleukins are produced mainly by white blood cells, and their job is to send signals out to other white blood cells telling them to report for duty. The name interleukins are easy to recall if you remember that the first part of the world 'inter' means between (communication between cells), and the second part, 'leukins,' refers to leukocytes, which is the technical name for white blood cells. Thus interleukins facilitate communication between white blood cells (leukocytes).

Chemokines initiate and promote inflammatory reactions. Chemokines are formed in response to cytokine activity. [42] Chemokines promote the localization and subsequent activation of immune cells at local tissue sites. These molecules play a major role

5. Markers of Immune Activity

in the successful clearing of viral and intracellular parasitic infections.

Complement System

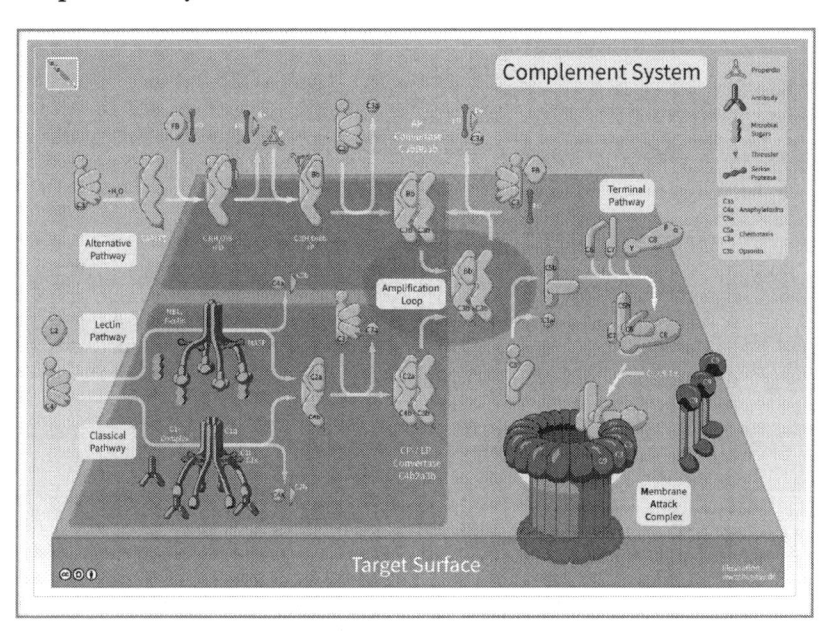

The complement system is an important part of our immune system and it has three different pathways that work together simultaneously:

- Classic pathway, which is part of adaptive immunity and is stimulated by antigen-antibody interactions.
- Alternative pathway, which is part of innate immunity and activates on contact with the cell surfaces of pathogens (lipopolysaccharides)
- Lectin pathway, which is also part of innate immunity and activates when it detects mannose sugars with are usually present on surfaces of infected cells.

Sometimes our immune system is able to eliminate an insult instantly, for example, when an antibody interacts with and causes

5. Markers of Immune Activity

the destruction of an antigen. Other times, the antibody does not precipitate the destruction of the antigen without additional help. In these instances, the binding of antibodies to antigen performs no immediately destructive function until it can activate an 'effector' mechanism. <u>The complement system serves that effector role.</u>

The complement system protects us in six ways: through "lysis" or breaking open the cells of an invader; by preparing for invader cell destruction by phagocytes; by amplifying inflammation; by moving toxic byproducts from the blood to the spleen and liver; by "complementing" the activity of T cells; and by aggregating virons, the infective form of a virus, for destruction.

Measuring Cytokines
It's important to know about cytokines and their action but it's challenging to actually measure them. Cytokines induce their biological effects at tiny pharmacological doses and have short half-lives. [43] Cytokines appearing in the blood are those not consumed at local sites or not rapidly removed from circulation. In general, the levels of many cytokines circulating in the blood of either healthy or diseased individuals are below the limit of detection by commercially available assays kits. The cytokine blood levels that can be measured may also show substantial variability because the values in the assays are at or near their limits of precise measurement. [44] In addition, blood levels of cytokines are susceptible to other factors such as patient behaviors, fasting, drugs, physical activity, blood collection, handling, processing, storage, as well as analytical techniques.

What to do? Fortunately, cytokines are <u>not</u> the end of the story. Other longer-lasting, common, and easily measured substances

5. Markers of Immune Activity

stimulated by cytokines persist in the blood long after cytokines have vanished. This brings us to the next chapter.

Chapter 6. Measuring My Immune Activity

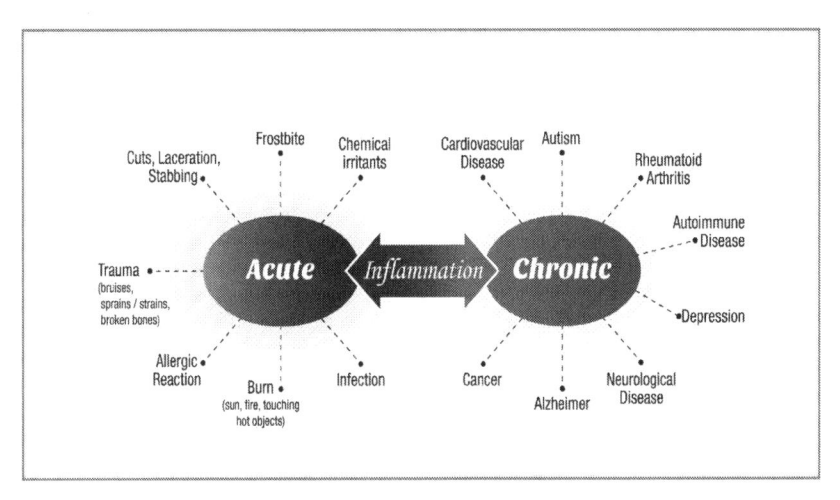

The activity of our immune system is complicated and elegant, yet the measurement of its activity is quite simple. Inflammation is the key response and inflammatory markers are both well known and highly correlated with immunity. Within the standard-of-care, inflammatory markers are often not considered, and if they are, normal values are for measuring an 'acute' (immediate) health condition. However, chronic inflammation is the key to understanding where we all lie on the **'health - disease continuum.'** If the goal is to prevent, identify and reverse early disease, our focus must be on measuring the smoldering fire, not the inferno. Chronic inflammation is persistent, low-grade inflammation that can last for years and in so doing is <u>the</u> sign of accelerated aging and disease. [45] [46] [47] [48] [49]

We have made understanding you chronic disease health and risk easy - by consolidating your important lab markers for inflammation into a single, highly intuitive value - your chronic disease temperature.

6. Measuring My Immune Activity

Chronic Disease Temperature™

Your Chronic Disease Temperature™ (CDT) is <u>the</u> measure of your risk for an early death! We created the CDT algorithm based on extensive research into diverse biomarkers as they related to premature mortality. In other words, when a given marker value showed a statistically validated increase of dying prematurely in populations. We start assigning a risk value at the lowest "abnormal" value. That is the first value that shows an increase in mortality.

Most everything in nature conforms to a log-linear scale. Think about driving your vehicle 30 mph, then accelerate to 60, then 90, then 120. Now you understand the concept of "log-linear." Chronic disease risk, as measured by biomarkers, also conform to a log-linear scale. Therefore, with <u>any</u> increase above the lowest abnormal lab value, your risk increases log-linearly. Our algorithm aggregates the risk from all of your inflammatory markers into a single number that is based on the measurement of your core body temperature. Anything above 98.6 in your CDT score signals an increased risk in mortality <u>and</u> morbidity. As you will see shortly, early mortality and early poor health are intimately connected. So your CDT is also your chronic disease barometer.

Combined biomarker risk scores have been proposed before but none have combined markers based on a single outcome. In the case of your CDT, that outcome just happens to be the most relevant to your health, early mortality risk. After all, isn't this what we are all hoping for - a longer and healthier life? It is well known, that people who die young of chronic conditions suffer many years of poor health. The figure on the next page, from a

6. Measuring My Immune Activity

study of longevity, illustrates the value of the CDT measurement in determining your current and future chronic health status.

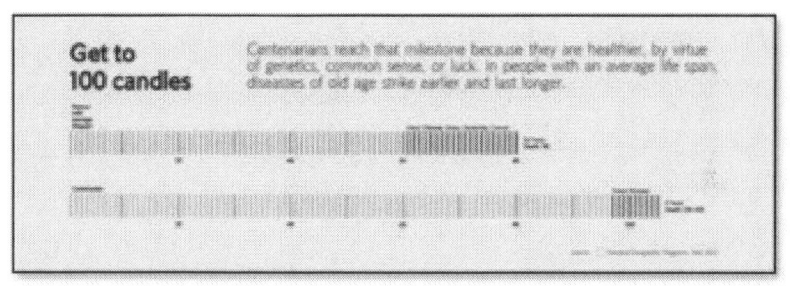

Get to 100 candles
Centenarians reach that milestone because they are healthier, by virtue of genetics, common sense, or luck. In people with an average life span, diseases of old age strike earlier and last longer.

This research clearly shows that people who live to 80 experience 19 years of declining health, log-linear, no doubt. Those who live to 100 only experience 9 years of declining health. Simply put, the longer you live - the longer you live a healthy life. People who live to 100 live 20 years longer than someone who dies at 80. More importantly, the person living to 100 experiences **30 more years of great health - a health span increased by 30 years.**

Let's dive into several markers of chronic inflammation that are evaluated in your CDT health score.

Homocysteine. This is a metabolic by-product of methionine metabolism. Progressively elevated blood levels of homocysteine are a documented risk marker for cardiovascular events and Alzheimer's disease. [50] Curiously, the standard-of-care continues to raise the upper limit of normal for homocysteine. It used to be around 12.5 mmol/L and now it is 15. However, many studies show an increase in all-cause and

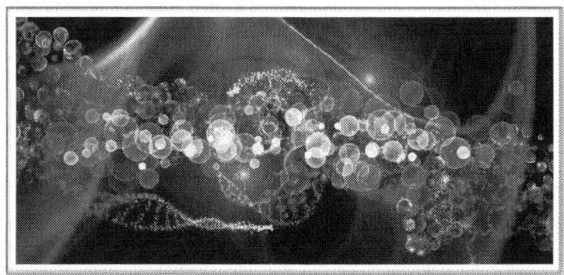

6. Measuring My Immune Activity

cardiovascular mortality at homocysteine levels significantly below these 'normal' values. [51] [52] Also interesting, the upper limit for cholesterol continues to go down. Note there is no drug available to lower homocysteine. Even slightly elevated levels of homocysteine (>6.3) can pose significant health risks, including damaging the lining of arteries and thickening blood. There are peer-reviewed studies showing a slight increase in mortality associated with slightly elevated homocysteine.

Most of the research looking at elevated homocysteine (Homocystinuria) and disease actually find stronger associations with aberrant methylation and folate metabolism abnormalities. Although homocysteine, by itself, at elevated levels is toxic, it may be an important marker of metabolic dysfunction and methylation disruption. [53]

As goes homocysteine levels, so goes your immune system. Homocysteine at elevated concentrations activates human monocytes and induces cytokine expression, amplifying the inflammatory response. [54] Homocysteine is also provided with immuno-modulating and pro-inflammatory activities. It enhances the production of cytokines such as IL-6, IL-8, and other immune cells thereby suggesting a possible additional role for homocysteine in the inflammatory process creating heart disease. [55]

Homocysteine is a much better predictor of your future health compared to cholesterol but cholesterol has a conveniently billable long-term drug treatment. And that treatment happens to be the biggest selling drug category of all time.

C-Reactive Protein (hsCRP or CRP). This is one of a number of acute phase reactant proteins that increases in response to inflammatory stimuli. We refer to the CRP value as a measure of

6. Measuring My Immune Activity

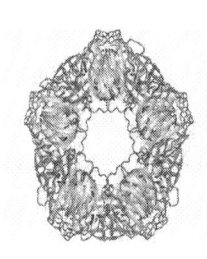

your chronic vascular (blood vessel) inflammation. Elevated CRP warns of many different conditions including cancer, cardiovascular disease, infection, diabetes, brain-related diseases from depression to Alzheimer's, and autoimmune diseases. Chronically elevated CRP, even as low as 0.6 micrograms per milliliter, is an indication of premature death from chronic disease. [56] [57] At the molecular level, production of CRP is induced by pro-inflammatory cytokines IL-1, IL-6, and IL-17 in the liver, showing the relationship between CRP and our immune response. [58]

No one parameter, including CRP, is accurate at assessing you chronic disease burden, but CRP is one of the most useful. In large epidemiological studies, elevated levels of CRP have been shown to be a strong indicator of heart and circulatory diseases and early mortality. Newer risk scores and biometric panels incorporate CRP including the Reynolds and Intermountain risk scores. These panels are seldom performed within the standard-of-care system.

Complete Blood Count with Differential (CBC w/diff).

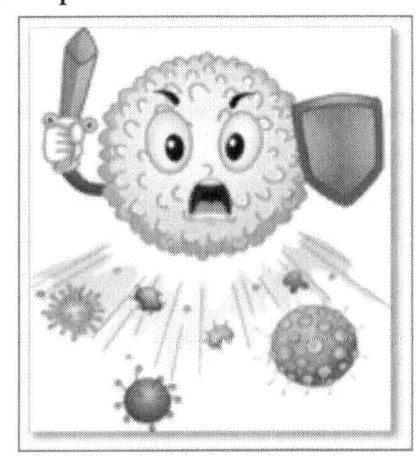

Measuring your complete blood count, with a particular focus on assessing white blood cell counts, gives a very accurate measure of both your innate and adaptive immune system activity. Total white blood cell counts alone are informative and highly predictive of your current and future chronic

6. Measuring My Immune Activity

health status. Harvard Medical School has recently asserted that "using the complete blood count risk score, an inexpensive tool that uses all of the information in the common blood test that includes information frequently underused. Physicians have used this CBC lab test for years, but they did not understand that all of its components provide information about life expectancy." [59]

Total white blood cell counts of just 6700 is an indication of premature death. "As part of the federally supported Women's Health Initiative, investigators at medical centers all over the United States collected information on 72,242 postmenopausal women 50 to 79 years old. All were free of heart and blood vessel disease at the start of the study. During six years of follow-up, 1,626 heart disease deaths, heart attacks, and strokes occurred. Women with more than 6.7 billion white cells per liter of blood (6,700 cells/mL) had more than double the risk of fatal heart disease than women with 4.7 billion cells per liter or lower (4,700 cells/mL). A count of 6,700 is considered to be normal, so what is "normal" may have to be redefined." [60] Note that the upper level of normal according to the standard-of-care is around 11,800 cells/mL! Wouldn't you like to know about your real risk for the #1 killer?

The CBC with differential blood test provides also provides great information about your immune system activity and health. This test includes values for the five different types of white blood cells, each with their own important function. The total white blood cell count, that includes each of the five subtypes, is a very powerful predictor of chronic disease and prognosis as indicated above. White blood cells protect the body against infection. If an infection develops, white blood cells attack and destroy the bacteria, virus, or other organisms. White blood cells are bigger than red blood cells but are fewer in number. When a person has a

6. Measuring My Immune Activity

bacterial infection, the number of white cells rises very quickly and will stay elevated, if only slightly, in the presence of chronic infection. The number of white blood cells is sometimes used to find an infection or to see how the body is dealing with cancer treatment or to determine if an immune system disorder exists. The optimal range for a healthy person relatively free of chronic disease is 4000-6000 cells/mL.

Neutrophil granulocytes. These are generally referred to as either neutrophils or polymorphonuclear neutrophils (or PMNs) and are subdivided into segmented neutrophils (or segs) and banded neutrophils (or bands). Neutrophils are the most abundant type of white blood cells in humans and other mammals, forming an essential part of the innate immune system. Neutrophils are recruited to the site of injury within minutes following trauma and are the hallmark of acute inflammation. These cells also protect the body against infection by destroying bacteria, thus are also a hallmark for chronic inflammation driven by bacterial infections.

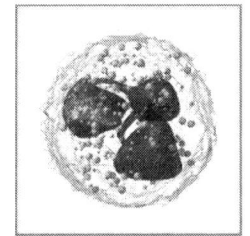

To better understand how predictive white blood cell counts, particularly neutrophils are regarding your future health, consider reading the works of Dr. Paul Ewald, an evolutionary biologist. Ewald states, "diseases we have long ascribed to genetic or environmental factors -- including some forms of heart disease, cancer, and mental illness -- are in many cases actually caused by infections." [61] Neutrophil counts, even well within normal values are a highly sensitive measure of chronic inflammation and bacterial infection. A single value may create a false positive because of an acute health issue, but chronically elevated neutrophils correlate strongly with poor health.

6. Measuring My Immune Activity

Eosinophil granulocytes. These are usually called eosinophils or, less commonly, acidophils and are a type of white blood cell. The functions of the eosinophil are varied, some of which are very similar to other white blood cells and they are also responsible for combating multicellular parasites and certain infections like mold. They also control mechanisms associated with allergy and asthma which are often tied to fungal infections. In addition, eosinophils may have a physiological role in organ formation.

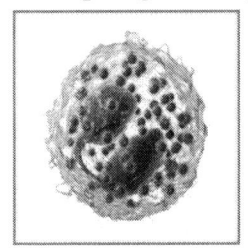

Parasitic infections are much more common than previously recognized especially today with so many people on acid-reducing drugs that dampen the gut immune system. Eosinophil levels need careful consideration. Toxoplasmosis is considered by the CDC one of a few high-priority but poorly recognized parasitic infections. Up to 60 million Americans may be infected by Toxoplasma Gondii. This parasite is able to penetrate the blood-brain barrier and contribute to mood disorders, Schizophrenia and even Alzheimer's.

Lymphocytes and Natural Killer (NK) Cells. NK cells are a part of the innate immune system and play a major role in defending the body from both tumors and virally infected cells. We are learning that viruses are the cause of many cancer cases, so appreciating your lymphocyte activity is extremely important to disease prevention. NK cells distinguish infected cells and tumors from normal cells by recognizing changes on the surface. NK cells are activated in response to a family of cytokines called interferons. Activated NK cells release cytotoxic (cell-killing) granules that then destroy the altered cells. They are named "natural killer cells" because of the

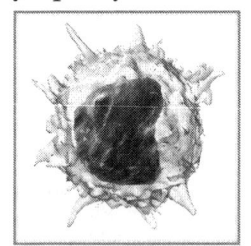

6. Measuring My Immune Activity

initial notion that they do not require prior activation in order to kill cells.

Your lymphocyte value is part of your CDT risk score by way of the neutrophil-to-lymphocyte ratio (NLR). This ratio is highly correlated to cardiovascular risk, cancer risk, and cancer prognosis. As part of your CDT result, we estimate your cancer risk using several highly related values included the NLR. Few practices use this ratio as a risk marker but hopefully, more doctors will study and report this important value to their patients in the near future. The good news is that you have full control over your NLR. We provide a solution to uncover your NLR and how to reduce it, in Chapter 7.

Basophils. They appear in many specific kinds of inflammatory reactions, particularly those that cause allergic symptoms. Like the other white blood cells, basophils are produced in the bone marrow but are found in many tissues throughout the body. Basophils contain anticoagulant heparin, which prevents blood from clotting too quickly. They also contain the vasodilator histamine, which promotes blood flow to tissues. They can be found in unusually high numbers at sites of infection, e.g., by ticks. Like eosinophils, basophils play a role in both parasitic infections and allergies. If your basophil level is low, it may be due to a severe allergic reaction. If you develop an infection, and your basophil levels are low, it may take longer to heal. In some cases, having too many basophils can result from certain blood cancers.

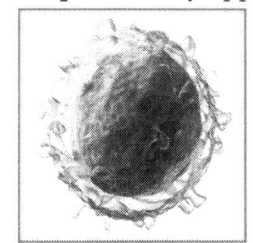

6. Measuring My Immune Activity

Monocytes. Monocytes are a type of white blood cell that fights off bacteria, viruses, and fungi. Monocytes are the biggest type of white blood cell in the immune system. Originally formed in the bone marrow, they are released into our blood and tissues. When certain germs enter the body, they quickly rush to the site for attack. Monocytes have the ability to change into another cell form called macrophages before facing the germs. They can actually consume harmful bacteria, fungi, and viruses. Then enzymes in the monocyte's body kill and break down the germs into pieces.

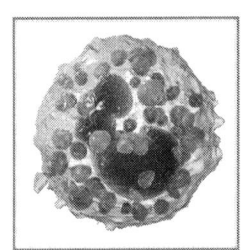

Monocytes help other white blood cells identify the type of germs that have invaded our body. After consuming the germs, the monocytes take parts of those germs, called antigens, and mount them outside their body like flags. Other white blood cells see the antigens and make antibodies designed to kill those specific types of germs. This is our adaptive immunity.

Vitamin D. This extremely important pro-hormone promotes calcium absorption in the gut and maintains adequate serum calcium and phosphate concentrations to enable normal mineralization of bone. It is also needed for bone growth and bone remodeling by osteoblasts and osteoclasts. Without sufficient vitamin D, bones can become thin, brittle, or misshapen. Vitamin D sufficiency prevents rickets in children and osteomalacia in adults. Vitamin D also helps protect older adults from osteoporosis. Vitamin D works in concert with Vitamin K2 in the directing of calcium out of our vessels (where calcium is harmful) and into our bones. Vitamin D has other roles in the body, including modulation of cell growth, neuromuscular and immune function, and reduction of inflammation.

6. Measuring My Immune Activity

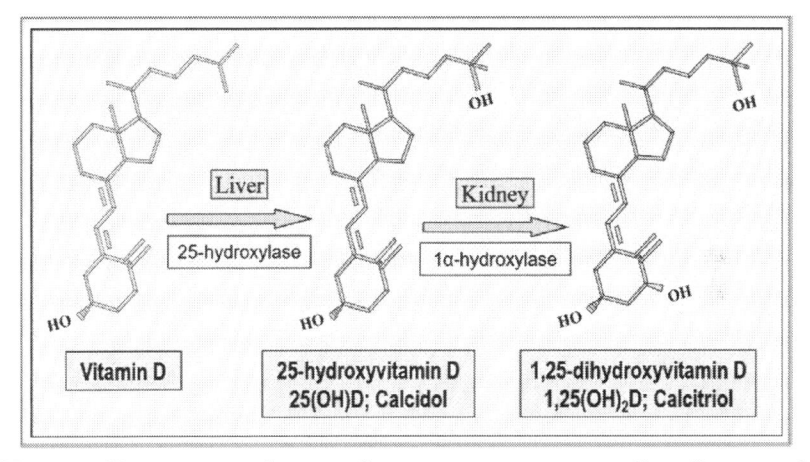

Vitamin D is a critical part of our immune system. It collects and is stored in our fat tissue. Like soldiers in their barracks, Vitamin D is always 'on the ready' to protect us from "insults" like an infection. When the immune system detects infection, like the soldiers who grab their weapons to respond, Vitamin D converts to the "activated" form. This activated form is now known to be antibiotic. The first hint of this "antibiotic" activity was noted over 150 years ago when people who took cod liver oil – which contains natural Vitamins D, A, and other fat-soluble vitamins – were somewhat protected from the scourge of tuberculosis.

Low vitamin D levels are associated with a higher prevalence of cancer, cardiovascular risk factors, and a higher risk of heart attack. A study of recent heart attack patients provided some patients with 4000 IU of vitamin D while others received no vitamin D. "A short course of treatment with vitamin D effectively attenuated the increase in circulating levels of inflammatory cytokines after an acute coronary event. Control group patients had increased cytokine and cellular adhesion molecules serum concentrations after 5 days, while the vitamin D-treated group had an attenuated elevation or a reduction of these parameters." [62] A supplemental dose of 4000 IU brings an individuals 25-hydroxyvitamin D

6. Measuring My Immune Activity

(blood) level to approximately 50 ng/ml. Our recommended range for vitamin D is 55 - 100 ng/ml. Don't be afraid to inform your medical professional that the limits being used for vitamin D are for bone health, not overall health.

Insulin. Abnormal fasting insulin, especially when combined with other risk factors, identifies patients at significantly higher risk for diabetes, heart, and circulatory diseases. Insulin is one of the most studied of all molecules in our bodies. Insulin rises before glucose or A1C in pre-diabetics and is thus a better biomarker for early detection of metabolic disorders.

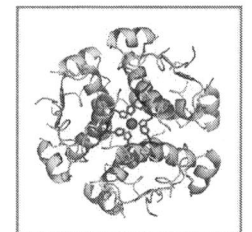

Fasting insulin level is arguably the most information-packed value for predicting metabolic syndrome but also for chronic disease risk in general. Chronically elevated insulin levels infer a cellular state of insulin resistance. It is considered as a pathological condition in which cells fail to respond normally to the hormone insulin. [63] To prevent hyperglycemia and noticeable organ damage over time from the inflammatory effects of elevated glucose, the body produces insulin in response to carbohydrate metabolism.

Under normal conditions of insulin sensitivity, this insulin response enables glucose to penetrate into body cells thereby allowing the concentration of glucose in the blood to achieve and maintain safe, non-inflammatory levels. In insulin resistance, pre-diabetes, and type 2 diabetes, insulin loses its effectiveness resulting in insulin, glucose, and triglycerides elevating dangerously and causing vascular inflammation to increase.

The clinical definition of insulin resistance does not adequately explain the root-cause of insulin-driven chronic disease. It is, however, a complex metabolic state impacted by society, brain chemistry, and emotional factors at the core. The simplest and most accurate description of chronically elevated insulin and insulin resistance is <u>malnutrition</u>.

Your Cells are Suffering from an Energy Crisis!

Did you know that it is possible for your cells to have plenty of calories yet still be starving? When cells are starved for nutrients, even with plenty of calories, we remain hungry. Governed by our brain, which in an effort to maintain our health, goes into self-preservation mode. The brain uses 10 times more energy compared to average cells in our body and has a high demand for repair and recover, which happens when we sleep. Recovery and repair are accomplished through nutrients, not just calories. [64] If we continue to feed our body low nutrient foods, a vicious cycle of hunger and insulin resistance is established. Our cell membranes "just say no" to more glucose fuel under these circumstances.

Two important disease-causing pathways are set up by insulin resistance: 1. cellular malnutrition and 2. inflammation. A consequence of cellular malnutrition and this includes immune cells, is poor repair and regeneration leading to both acute and chronic disease susceptibility. Inflammation from excess circulating glucose and hormones leads to oxidative stress and damage to tissue, exacerbating the effects of cellular malnutrition. The solution to this conundrum is quite simple, always consume foods high in nutrient density.
Next time your doctor orders a blood draw, demand a fasting insulin test. Your ideal number is 2-6 mIU/L.

6. Measuring My Immune Activity

Fibrinogen. This is a plasma glycoprotein that is involved in clotting response to an injury. Thus, fibrinogen rises in the presence of cuts and acute trauma. However, it also elevates slightly and steadily in response to chronic vascular inflammation. Individuals with elevated CRP (vessel inflammation) and RDW (red blood cell distribution width) often have an elevated fibrinogen level - reflecting repair of damaged endothelial tissue inside vessel walls. Cytokines, both protective and inflammatory, track with levels of fibrinogen in blood making it an excellent marker for measuring immune system activity. [65] Ideal fibrinogen levels are between 175 and 285 mg/dL.

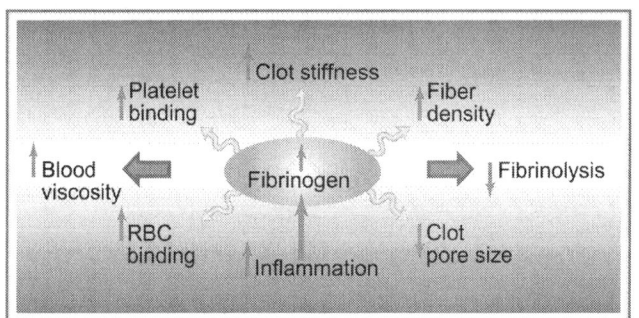

The combination of elevated fibrinogen and other cardiovascular risk factors such as CRP signals substantially increased disease potential. This does not imply that fibrinogen is a therapeutic target, rather it's part of the immune response to damage for the purposes of repair.

ESR or SED rate. SED rate is an important test that measures how fast red blood cell platelets settle. It is used to detect chronic inflammation associated with infections, autoimmune disorders, and cancer. The platelet settling rate depends on red blood cell (RBC) mass, volume, and shape; electrostatic (charge) electrical forces; and the protein constitution of plasma. Electrostatic forces normally cause RBCs to repel each other and inhibit their aggregation. An increased amount of plasma fibrinogen or

6. Measuring My Immune Activity

globulins coat the RBCs, foster their aggregation, and hasten settling, consequently elevating the ESR.

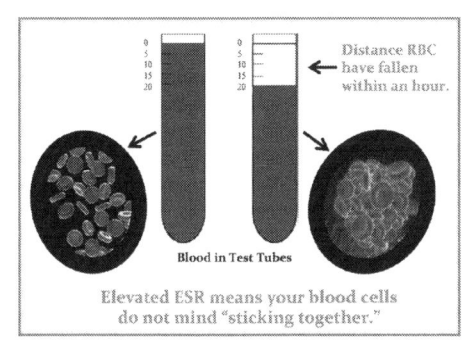

Healthy blood cells in a healthy, inflammation-free body, hold a negative charge and SED rate is a way to estimate the relative charge on and health of the cell platelets. Fast sedimentation implies low (poor) charge on the blood cells and is associated with higher levels of inflammation and early mortality.

SED rate is significantly and positively correlated with markers of inflammatory immune activation and is also a marker of infectious processes. [66] [67]

Ferritin. Checking your iron levels is done through a blood test called a serum ferritin test. The study of iron in the human brain is particularly important in the context of Alzheimer's disease. Iron is both essential for healthy brain function and is implicated as a factor in neurodegeneration. The chemical form of the iron is particularly critical, as this affects its toxicity and disrupted iron metabolism is linked to regional iron accumulation and pathological hallmarks, such as senile plaques and neurofibrillary tangles. Men should generally avoid iron supplementation.

Uric Acid. Uric acid is recognized as a marker of gout as well as being a major natural antioxidant, prohibiting the occurrence of cellular damage. [68] According to some research, "Notwithstanding the associated increased risk of cardiovascular disease, higher levels of uric acid are associated with a decreased risk of dementia and

6. Measuring My Immune Activity

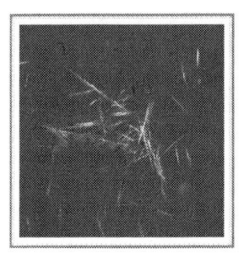

better cognitive function later in life."[69] A high level of serum uric acid was found to predict the development of hypertension, obesity, insulin resistance, kidney disease, and cardiovascular events. [70][71][72][73] A potential mechanism by which uric acid could be associated with cardiovascular morbidity is via inflammation. [74][75]

Uric acid levels assist in measuring immune system activity. Its levels are associated positively with IL-6, CRP, and TNF-α and negatively with IL-1β. The current normal lab values, on the high end of uric acid, are for gout. However, according to very recent research, "compared to inflammatory markers such as CRP and IL-6 serum uric acid levels may predict future CVD risk in patients with stable CHD with a risk increase even at levels considered normal."[76]

Uric acid remains an important test that should be performed routinely to measure health and health trends. It is a key marker for systemic hypoxia (lack of oxygen). Athletes often have high uric acid after exercise as do mountaineers. Ideal normal uric acid levels are between 5 and 6 mg/dL.

Red Blood Cell Distribution Width (RDW). Did you know that the diameter of a red blood cell is greater than the diameter of a capillary - the tiny vessels of your circulatory system? This means that your red blood cells must elongate to "squeeze" through them - like a worm working its way through the soil. [77] Doctors view red blood cell distribution width (RDW) as a measure of anemia. However, that is only a small part of the story. This measurement, often ignored in the standard of care, is a profound measurement

6. Measuring My Immune Activity

of your current health risk and future health prognosis. A complete blood cell count with differential includes the RDW data. Some labs are not publishing this data because doctors don't want it included in the reports. Thus the RDW becomes one less thing to explain. It is disappearing in the major medical websites like Mayo and WebMd too.

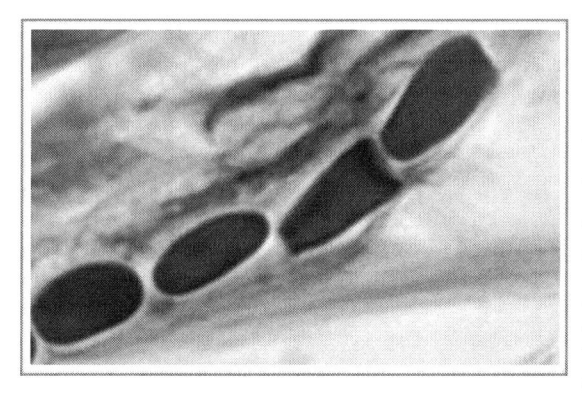

RDW needs to re-emerge as an indicator because of its predictive value for chronic diseases, with cardiovascular diseases leading the list. A PubMed search that includes the term "red blood cell distribution width," in the "title only" yielded 349 articles. Many of the articles discuss the association between RDW and disease. About 42% of the articles tied abnormal RDW and cardiovascular diseases and 15% associated abnormal RDW with early mortality. [78] [79]

A Harvard Medical School and Harvard School of Public Health team published, "Red blood cell distribution width and mortality risk in a community-based prospective cohort." Their conclusion is pretty clear: "Higher RDW was associated with increased mortality risk in this large, community-based sample, an association not specific to CVD. Study of elevated RDW may, therefore, yield novel pathophysiological insights, and measurement of RDW may contribute to risk assessment." They also state: "..the highest quintile of RDW, compared with the lowest, was significantly associated with 134% increased risk of CV mortality after multivariable adjustment" and "..the highest quintile of RDW,

6. Measuring My Immune Activity

compared with the lowest, was significantly associated with <u>an 88% increased risk of death due to cancer</u>." [80]

For a more complete explanation of RDW, read "Quarterback Your Own Health - How to Take and Lower Your Chronic Disease Temperature. [81] Your target RDW is <12.5%

Eye Diseases. Amyloidosis as a marker of infection was discussed in Chapter 2. The most convenient place in our body to screen for amyloid in our eyes. A little-known fact is that eye diseases are a sign of a deadly underlying cardiovascular disease. People diagnosed with cataracts, a form of amyloidosis, die at **10 times** the rate compared to people diagnosed with either breast or prostate cancer. The death rate is 11% in 6 years according to a major NIH study called AREDS (Age-Related Eye Disease Study). [82] Similar poor outcomes occur for people diagnosed with macular degeneration and glaucoma. Macular degeneration is also a disease with amyloid formations, called Drusen.

When amyloid formation occurs in your eye, biomarkers for inflammation also rise. [83] Age-related macular degeneration (AMD) and cardiovascular disease share common risk factors. Inflammatory biomarkers, including CRP, interleukin 6 and soluble tumor necrosis factor. High CRP is a well-known risk factor for future cataract formation - and by extension - high cardiovascular mortality. Do you know if you have high levels of inflammation in your body as measured by CRP? If you have a cataract forming or if you had cataract surgery, you can be sure your CRP is most likely up as are other chronic immune activation markers. For an extensive review of your eye as <u>the best</u> screening tool for your future health, read "Quarterback Your Own Health - How to Take and Lower Your Chronic Disease Temperature." [84]

6. Measuring My Immune Activity

Eye Diseases are DEADLY Diseases.

The Chronic Disease Temperature™ (CDT) health risk scale combines existing and emerging concepts for improving the evaluation of disease risk and measurement of active chronic disease. Every marker in this chapter, and additional ones not discussed here are included in the CDT scales. Arguably the most important asset provided by your total CDT score is our ability to determine if you have a low-grade infection like Lyme (Borrelia Burgdorferi) or other treatable intracellular pathogens that are currently producing a low-grade immune response, inflammation, and chronic disease today.

The significant attributes of the CDT scale are:
1. Consideration of multiple biomarkers
2. Selection of indicators based on traditional and new predictive tools based on inflammaging and the allostatic load
3. Harmonizing each marker to a standard endpoint – increase in early mortality risk
4. Consideration of risk contribution based on log-linear scales appropriate for each biomarker using hazard ratios for mortality
5. Combination of the risk values from each marker into a single number score for ease of understanding and comparison of trends

The aggregate CDT score is an indicator of early mortality and associated morbidity, while the values for each marker reflect both mortality risk and disease risk based on the association of a given marker to disease. This single number is intended to be an important bridge to better health decisions as most patients do not

6. Measuring My Immune Activity

understand the meaning of their current lab values. [85] The CDT does not constitute a medical diagnosis of disease any more than does any individual marker, like homocysteine, but does statistically afford better predictive capability and measurement of disease progression or regression.

Who should measure their CDT? Answer: Anyone interested in knowing their current and future health status - in great detail - and also want to be able to track their progress towards achieving better health and a longer life.

If You Are Not Measuring, You ARE Guessing

Chapter 7. Live Longer & Healthier

If you are not measuring - you're guessing. In a world full of fads and unsubstantiated trends, isn't it time to know YOU? The way to know if you are doing the right thing is to measure yourself thoroughly and accurately, make the appropriate adjustment, and then measure yourself again. There is no other way to know if you are doing the right things for you.

We have designed a **3-STEP** program to achieve your health goals. It all starts with measurement. First, ponder this quote by one of the top 3 medical doctors of all time - Claude Bernard of 19th Century France who is the father of experimental medicine:

> "The experimenter who does not know what he is looking for
> will not understand what he finds."

Step 1: Measure Your Chronic Life Risks

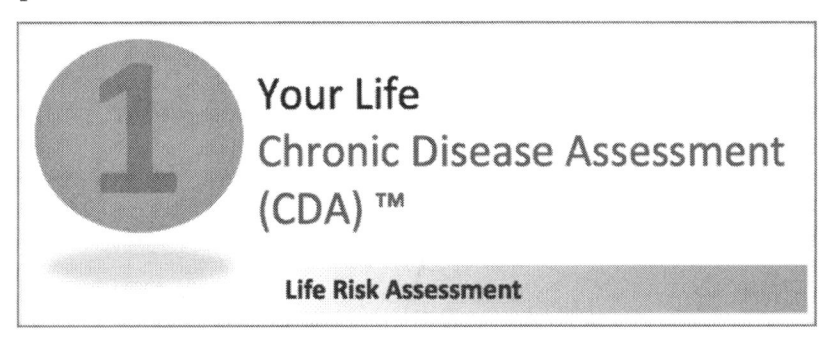

Your Life
Chronic Disease Assessment (CDA) ™

Life Risk Assessment

This life assessment is a questionnaire built by our Harvard Medical School colleagues and incorporates the best of Functional Medicine. The full assessment includes 120 questions and takes about 30 minutes to complete. You can also take the "FREE Risk

7. Live Longer & Healthier

at a Glance Quiz" found on our website home page (https://www.healthrevivalpartners.com/). However, this is a 'mini' version and far less accurate assessment.

To take the entire assessment and receive a 1-hr consultation to review your results and begin a path to better longevity, visit: https://www.healthrevivalpartners.com/shop

Step 2: Measure Your Chronic Disease Risk
This biometric panel, built by our Harvard Medical School colleagues, and compiled by our MIT-trained medical scientist incorporates over $2,500,000,000,000 of medical research. It combines high sensitivity and a broad array of relevant and important biomarkers into a single health score.

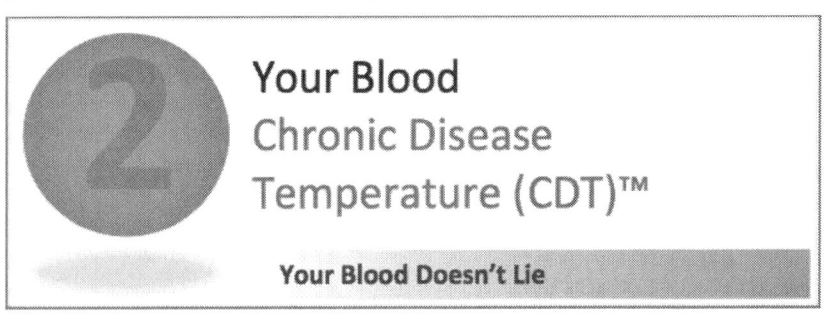

Your Blood
Chronic Disease Temperature (CDT)™

Your Blood Doesn't Lie

Where do you lie on the
health - disease continuum?

Get your CDT and remove all doubts.

7. Live Longer & Healthier

To obtain your Chronic Disease Temperature™, get our complimentary comprehensive report, and a consultation with either one of our doctors or the panel developer, visit: https://www.healthrevivalpartners.com/shop

Individualized Health Revival Plan

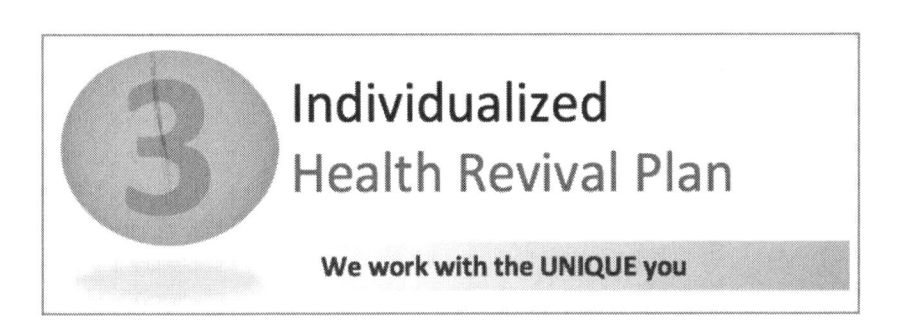

We work with the UNIQUE you

Step 3: Craft and Implement your 'Health Revival' Plan
We make getting and staying healthy easy because we recognize that it's not about a couple of big, unmanageable things - it's all about the little things. We measure your health accurately - at the root-cause level of disease. Next, we partner up to implement a plan aimed at overcoming the many little things that may be holding you back. Your body is a symphony and all the 'musicians and instruments' contribute to the magnificence of the symphonic sound of health.

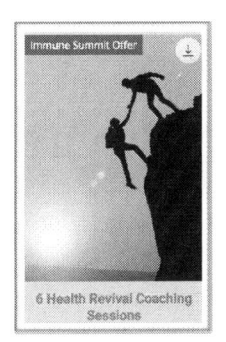

To start your personal health revival program visit:
https://www.healthrevivalpartners.com/shop

Experience **P4R** Medicine (Predictive, Preventive, Personalized, Participatory and Reversible) at it's best.

7. Live Longer & Healthier

Join the Health Revival Movement!

Dr. Lewis

About the Author
Dr. Thomas J. Lewis is a Medical Scientist. He holds a Ph.D. in Chemistry from MIT and certification from the Harvard School of Public Health. He is an entrepreneur and healthcare professional with expertise in toxic substances, drug development, biotechnology, health technology, and medical protocol development. For the past decades he has worked closely with senior researchers and clinicians at Harvard Medical School and has developed a program for chronic disease root cause prevention, screening, diagnosis, and treatment. Alzheimer's disease and the most serious eye diseases, macular degeneration and glaucoma have been a particular focus.

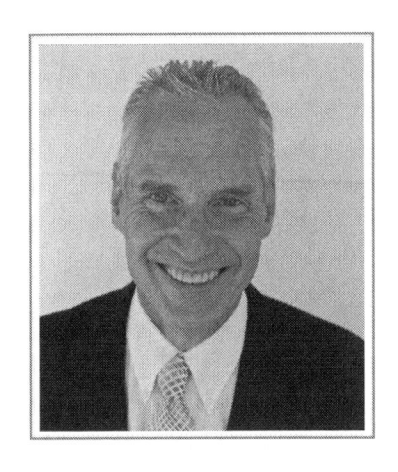

Dr. Lewis opened the first-of-its-kind Alzheimer's prevention, screening, early detection, and treatment center in the Orlando, Florida area in 2014. He works closely with Dr. Clement Trempe, 41 years at Harvard Medical School who is one of few doctors in the world who treats chronic eye diseases as systemic inflammatory conditions – and reverses these conditions with great success. It was through this work that Dr. Trempe developed his protocol for diagnosing, treating, and reversing Alzheimer's disease that is now an integral part of the Health Revival offering.

Dr. Lewis has written two books: "The End of Alzheimer's – The Brain and Beyond," (2nd Ed.) and "Quarterback Your Own Health – How to Take and Lower Your Chronic Disease Temperature."

Dr. Lewis

He has several patents and numerous publications. The most recent patent involves the identification and use of both physiological and pathological biomarkers that are able to accurately predict future morbidity (disease) and mortality. This risk is presented by way of a single risk value coined your "Chronic Disease Temperature™. He has also created a software-based medical intake form that is designed to determine the current and future risk of accelerated aging and chronic disease in individuals.

References:

[1] Hooper, Judith, and Paul Ewald. "A New Germ Theory." The Atlantic, Atlantic Media Company, 1 Feb. 1999, www.theatlantic.com/magazine/archive/1999/02/a-new-germ-theory/377430/.

[2] Allison, James, and Tasuku Honjo. "The Nobel Prize in Physiology or Medicine 2018." Nobelprize.org, Nobel Prize Committee, 21 Oct. 2018, www.nobelprize.org/prizes/medicine/2018/press-release/.

[3] Bissell, M. J., & Hines, W. C. (2011). Why don't we get more cancer? A proposed role of the microenvironment in restraining cancer progression. *Nature medicine, 17*(3), 320.

[4] Son, D. J., Lee, J. W., Lee, Y. H., Song, H. S., Lee, C. K., & Hong, J. T. (2007). Therapeutic application of anti-arthritis, pain-releasing, and anti-cancer effects of bee venom and its constituent compounds. Pharmacology & therapeutics, 115(2), 246-270.

[5] Fortier, L. A., McCarrel, T. M., Sundman, E. A., Schnabel, L. V., Cole, B. J., Boswell, S., & Karas, V. (2011). Biologic Therapy for Joint Disease Platelet-Rich Plasma, Interleukin-1 Receptor Antagonist Protein/Autologous Condition Serum, and Bone Marrow Aspirate. In Proceedings of the Annual Convention of the American Association of Equine Practitioners (San Antonio, EUA,).

[6] Ray-Coquard I, Cropet C, Van Glabbeke M, et al. Lymphopenia as a prognostic factor for overall survival in advanced carcinomas, sarcomas, and lymphomas. Cancer Res. 2009;69(13):5383-91.

[7] Alberts, B., Johnson, A., Lewis, J., Walter, P., Raff, M., & Roberts, K. (2002). Molecular Biology of the Cell 4th Edition: International Student Edition.

[8] (2017). The Importance of Cholesterol in Psychopathology: A Review of Recent Contributions. Indian journal of psychological medicine, 39(2), 109-113.

[9] Ravnskov, U. (2003). High cholesterol may protect against infections and atherosclerosis. Qjm, 96(12), 927-934.

[10] Ravnskov, U., Diamond, D. M., Hama, R., Hamazaki, T., Hammarskjöld, B., Hynes, N., ... & McCully, K. S. (2016). Lack of an association or an inverse association between low-density-lipoprotein cholesterol and mortality in the elderly: a systematic review. BMJ open, 6(6), e010401.

[11] Claxton, Ami J., et al. "Association between serum total cholesterol and HIV infection in a high-risk cohort of young men." JAIDS Journal of Acquired Immune Deficiency Syndromes 17.1 (1998): 51-57.

[12] Marquart, M. E., Monds, K. S., McCormick, C. C., Dixon, S. N., Sanders, M. E., Reed, J. M., ... & O'Callaghan, R. J. (2007). Cholesterol as treatment for pneumococcal keratitis: cholesterol-specific inhibition of pneumolysin in the cornea. Investigative ophthalmology & visual science, 48(6), 2661-2666.

[13] Albert-Ludwigs-Universität Freiburg. (2012, December 21). Cholesterol boosts the memory of the immune system. ScienceDaily. Retrieved November 5, 2018 from www.sciencedaily.com/releases/2012/12/121221081619.htm

[14] U. Ravnskov; High cholesterol may protect against infections and atherosclerosis, QJM: An International Journal of Medicine, Volume 96, Issue 12, 1 December 2003, Pages 927–934, https://doi.org/10.1093/qjmed/hcg150

[15] Ravnskov, U., & McCully, K. S. (2009). Vulnerable plaque formation from obstruction of vasa vasorum by homocysteinylated and oxidized lipoprotein aggregates complexed with microbial remnants and LDL autoantibodies. Annals of Clinical & Laboratory Science, 39(1), 3-16.

[16] Deans, E., (2018, March 11). Cholesterol and Suicide (Again). Psychology Today. Retrieved October 1, 2018 from https://www.psychologytoday.com/us/blog/evolutionary-psychiatry/201803/low-cholesterol-and-suicide-again.

[17] Petursson, H., Sigurdsson, J. A., Bengtsson, C., Nilsen, T. I., & Getz, L. (2012). Is the use of cholesterol in mortality risk algorithms in clinical guidelines valid? Ten years prospective data from the Norwegian HUNT 2 study. Journal of evaluation in clinical practice, 18(1), 159-168.

[18] Weverling-Rijnsburger, Annelies WE, et al. "Total cholesterol and risk of mortality in the oldest old." The Lancet 350.9085 (1997): 1119-1123.

[19] Mehta D, Jackson R, Paul G, Shi J, Sabbagh M. Why do trials for Alzheimer's disease drugs keep failing? A discontinued drug perspective for 2010-2015. Expert Opin Investig Drugs. 2017;26(6):735-739.

[20] Kagan BL, Jang H, Capone R, et al. Antimicrobial properties of amyloid peptides. Mol Pharm. 2011;9(4):708-17.

[21] Soscia, S. J., Kirby, J. E., Washicosky, K. J., Tucker, S. M., Ingelsson, M., Hyman, B., ... & Moir, R. D. (2010). The Alzheimer's disease-associated amyloid β-protein is an antimicrobial peptide. PloS one, 5(3), e9505.

[22] Kumar DK, Choi SH, Washicosky KJ, et al. Amyloid-β peptide protects against microbial infection in mouse and worm models of Alzheimer's disease. Sci Transl Med. 2016;8(340):340ra72.

[23] Goldstein, L. E., Muffat, J. A., Cherny, R. A., Moir, R. D., Ericsson, M. H., Huang, X., ... & Masters, C. L. (2003). Cytosolic β-amyloid deposition and supranuclear cataracts in lenses from people with Alzheimer's disease. The Lancet, 361(9365), 1258-1265.

[24] Soscia, S. J., Kirby, J. E., Washicosky, K. J., Tucker, S. M., Ingelsson, M., Hyman, B., ... & Moir, R. D. (2010). The Alzheimer's disease-associated amyloid β-protein is an antimicrobial peptide. PloS one, 5(3), e9505.
Noble, D. (2008). Claude Bernard, the first systems biologist, and the future of physiology. Experimental Physiology, 93(1), 16-26.

[26] Oldstone, M. B. A. (1989). Molecular mimicry as a mechanism for the cause and as a probe uncovering etiologic agent (s) of autoimmune disease. In Molecular Mimicry (pp. 127-135). Springer, Berlin, Heidelberg.

[27] Families Say Lexington Nutrition Health Coach Can Cure Deadly Food Allergies. (2017, May 15). Retrieved from https://boston.cbslocal.com/2017/05/15/food-allergies-lexington-nutrition-health-coach-lombardo-amy-thieringer/

[28] Feed Your Kids Peanuts, Early and Often, New Guidelines Urge. (2017, December 22). Retrieved from https://www.nytimes.com/2017/01/05/well/eat/feed-your-kids-peanuts-early-and-often-new-guidelines-urge.html

[29] Selgrade MK, Cooper GS, Germolec DR, Heindel JJ. Linking environmental agents and autoimmune disease: an agenda for future research. Environ Health Perspect. 1999;107(Suppl. 5):811–3

[30] Ercolini, A. M., & Miller, S. D. (2009). The role of infections in autoimmune disease. Clinical and experimental immunology, 155(1), 1-15.

[31] Imhann, F., Bonder, M. J., Vila, A. V., Fu, J., Mujagic, Z., Vork, L., ... & Dijkstra, G. (2016). Proton pump inhibitors affect the gut microbiome. Gut, 65(5), 740-748.

[32] Imhann, F., Vich Vila, A., Bonder, M. J., Lopez Manosalva, A. G., Koonen, D. P., Fu, J., ... & Weersma, R. K. (2017). The influence of proton pump inhibitors and other commonly used medication on the gut microbiota. Gut microbes, 8(4), 351-358.

[33] Risk of Inflammatory Bowel Disease with Oral Contraceptives and Menopausal Hormone Therapy: Current Evidence and Future Directions. Drug Saf. 2016;39(3):193-7.

[34] Nature Microbiology. (2018, March 19). Gut microbes are vulnerable to wide range of drugs. Retrieved from https://www.nature.com/articles/d41586-018-02780-x

[35] Severance EG, Yolken RH, Eaton WW. Autoimmune diseases, gastrointestinal disorders and the microbiome in schizophrenia: more than a gut feeling. Schizophr Res. 2014;176(1):23-35.

[36] Sachdeva, A., Cannon, C. P., Deedwania, P. C., LaBresh, K. A., Smith Jr, S. C., Dai, D., ... & Fonarow, G. C. (2009). Lipid levels in patients hospitalized with coronary artery disease: an analysis of 136,905 hospitalizations in Get With The Guidelines. American heart journal, 157(1), 111-117.

[37] Claus, M., Dychus, N., Ebel, M., Damaschke, J., Maydych, V., Wolf, O. T., ... & Watzl, C. (2016). Measuring the immune system: a comprehensive approach for the analysis of immune functions in humans. Archives of toxicology, 90(10), 2481-2495.

[38] Brodin, P., & Davis, M. M. (2016). Human immune system variation. Nature reviews. Immunology, 17(1), 21-29.
[39] Lewis, Thomas J. "Disease Mitigation and Elimination Health Learning Engine." U.S. Patent Application No. 15/667,297.
[40] Enroth, S., Johansson, Å., Enroth, S. B., & Gyllensten, U. (2014). Strong effects of genetic and lifestyle factors on biomarker variation and use of personalized cutoffs. Nature communications, 5, 4684.
[41] Lunney, J. K. (1998). Cytokines orchestrating the immune response. Revue scientifique et technique-Office international des épizooties, 17, 84-89.
[42] Oppenheim J.J., Zachariae C.O.C., Mukaida W. & Matsushima K. (1991). - Properties of the novel proinflammatory supergene intercrine cytokine family. Annu. Rev. Immunol, 9, 617-638.
[43] Whiteside TL. Cytokine assays. Biotechniques. 2002;33:S4–S15
[44] Fahey, J. L. (1998). Cytokines, plasma immune activation markers, and clinically relevant surrogate markers in human immunodeficiency virus infection. Clinical and diagnostic laboratory immunology, 5(5), 597-603.
[45] Franceschi, C., & Campisi, J. (2014). Chronic inflammation (inflammaging) and its potential contribution to age-associated diseases. Journals of Gerontology Series A: Biomedical Sciences and Medical Sciences, 69(Suppl_1), S4-S9.
[46] Laimer, M., Ebenbichler, C. F., Kaser, S., Sandhofer, A., Weiss, H., Nehoda, H., ... & Patsch, J. R. (2002). Markers of chronic inflammation and obesity: a prospective study on the reversibility of this association in middle-aged women undergoing weight loss by surgical intervention. International journal of obesity, 26(5), 659.
[47] Festa, A., D'Agostino Jr, R., Williams, K., Karter, A. J., Mayer-Davis, E. J., Tracy, R. P., & Haffner, S. M. (2001). The relation of body fat mass and distribution to markers of chronic inflammation. International journal of obesity, 25(10), 1407.
[48] Wu, T. L., Chang, P. Y., Tsao, K. C., Sun, C. F., Wu, L. L., & Wu, J. T. (2007). A panel of multiple markers associated with chronic systemic inflammation and the risk of atherogenesis is detectable in asthma and chronic obstructive pulmonary disease. Journal of clinical laboratory analysis, 21(6), 367-371.
[49] Buchwald, D., Wener, M. H., Pearlman, T., & Kith, P. (1997). Markers of inflammation and immune activation in chronic fatigue and chronic fatigue syndrome. The Journal of rheumatology, 24(2), 372-376.
[50] McCully, K. S. (2015). Homocysteine metabolism, atherosclerosis, and diseases of aging. Compr physiol, 6(1), 471-505.
[51] Peng, H. Y., Man, C. F., Xu, J., & Fan, Y. (2015). Elevated homocysteine levels and risk of cardiovascular and all-cause mortality: a meta-analysis of prospective studies. Journal of Zhejiang University-SCIENCE B, 16(1), 78-86.

[52] Peng, H. Y., Man, C. F., Xu, J., & Fan, Y. (2015). Elevated homocysteine levels and risk of cardiovascular and all-cause mortality: a meta-analysis of prospective studies. Journal of Zhejiang University-SCIENCE B, 16(1), 78-86.
[53] Pizzorno, J. (2014). Homocysteine: Friend or Foe?. Integrative Medicine: A Clinician's Journal, 13(4), 8.
[54] Su, S. J., Huang, L. W., Pai, L. S., Liu, H. W., & Chang, K. L. (2005). Homocysteine at pathophysiologic concentrations activates human monocyte and induces cytokine expression and inhibits macrophage migration inhibitory factor expression. Nutrition, 21(10), 994-1002.
[55] Lazzerini, P. E., Selvi, E., Lorenzini, S., Capecchi, P. L., Ghittoni, R., Bisogno, S., ... & Laghi-Pasini, F. (2006). Homocysteine enhances cytokine production in cultured synoviocytes from rheumatoid arthritis patients. Clinical and experimental rheumatology, 24(4), 387.
[56] Mendall, M. A., Strachan, D. P., Butland, B. K., Ballam, L., Morris, J., Sweetnam, P. M., & Elwood, P. C. (2000). C-reactive protein: relation to total mortality, cardiovascular mortality and cardiovascular risk factors in men. European Heart Journal, 21(19), 1584-1590.
[57] Harris, T. B., Ferrucci, L., Tracy, R. P., Corti, M. C., Wacholder, S., Ettinger Jr, W. H., ... & Wallace, R. (1999). Associations of elevated Interleukin-6 and C-Reactive protein levels with mortality in the elderly*. The American journal of medicine, 106(5), 506-512.
[58] Eklund, C. M. (2009). Proinflammatory cytokines in CRP baseline regulation. Advances in clinical chemistry, 48, 111-136.
[59] Intermountain Medical Center. (2018, November 16). New study helps predict life expectancy using complete blood count risk score. Retrieved from https://www.sciencedaily.com/releases/2013/11/131119100931.htm
[60] Mason, J - Harvard Medical School, (2005, April 5). Simple test predicts heart attack risk. Retrieved from https://www.worldhealth.net/news/simple_test_predicts_heart_attack_risk/
[61] Hooper, J. (1999, February). A New Germ Theory. Retrieved from https://www.theatlantic.com/magazine/archive/1999/02/a-new-germ-theory/377430/
[62] Arnson, Y., Itzhaky, D., Mosseri, M., Barak, V., Tzur, B., Agmon-Levin, N., & Amital, H. (2013). Vitamin D inflammatory cytokines and coronary events: a comprehensive review. Clinical reviews in allergy & immunology, 45(2), 236-247.
[63] American Diabetes Association. (2014). Diagnosis and classification of diabetes mellitus. Diabetes care, 37(Supplement 1), S81-S90.
[64] Swaminathan, N. (2008, April 29). Why Does the Brain Need So Much Power? Retrieved from https://www.scientificamerican.com/article/why-does-the-brain-need-s/

[65] Vasse, M., Paysant, J., Soria, J., Collet, J. P., Vannier, J. P., & Soria, C. (1996). Regulation of fibrinogen biosynthesis by cytokines, consequences on the vascular risk. Pathophysiology of Haemostasis and Thrombosis, 26(Suppl. 4), 331-339.

[66] S.D Anker, K Egerer, H.-D Volk, W.J Kox, P.A Poole-Wilson, A.J.S Coats. Elevated soluble CD14 receptors and altered cytokines in chronic heart failure. Am J Cardiol, 79 (1997), pp. 1426-1430.

[67] Sharma, R., Rauchhaus, M., Ponikowski, P. P., Varney, S., Poole-Wilson, P. A., Mann, D. L., ... & Anker, S. D. (2000). The relationship of the erythrocyte sedimentation rate to inflammatory cytokines and survival in patients with chronic heart failure treated with angiotensin-converting enzyme inhibitors. Journal of the American College of Cardiology, 36(2), 523-528.

[68] Martinon F, Petrilli V, Mayor A, Tardivel A, Tschopp J (2006) Gout-associated uric acid crystals activate the NALP3 inflammasome. Nature 440: 237–241

[69] Euser, S. M., Hofman, A., Westendorp, R. G. J., & Breteler, M. M. (2008). Serum uric acid and cognitive function and dementia. Brain, 132(2), 377-382.

[70] Alper AB Jr, Chen W, Yau L, Srinivasan SR, Berenson GS, et al. (2005) Childhood uric acid predicts adult blood pressure: the Bogalusa Heart Study. Hypertension 45: 34–38.

[71] Johnson RJ, Kang DH, Feig D, Kivlighn S, Kanellis J, et al. (2003) Is there a pathogenetic role for uric acid in hypertension and cardiovascular and renal disease? Hypertension 41: 1183–1190.

[72] Bonora E, Targher G, Zenere MB, Saggiani F, Cacciatori V, et al. (1996) Relationship of uric acid concentration to cardiovascular risk factors in young men. Role of obesity and central fat distribution. The Verona Young Men Atherosclerosis Risk Factors Study. Int J Obes Relat Metab Disord 20: 975–980.

[73] Ogura T, Matsuura K, Matsumoto Y, Mimura Y, Kishida M, et al. (2004) Recent trends of hyperuricemia and obesity in Japanese male adolescents, 1991 through 2002. Metabolism 53: 448–453.

[74] Manzato E (2007) Uric acid: an old actor for a new role. Intern Emerg Med 2: 1–2.

[75] Montalcini T, Gorgone G, Gazzaruso C, Sesti G, Perticone F, et al. (2007) Relation between serum uric acid and carotid intima-media thickness in healthy postmenopausal women. Intern Emerg Med 2: 19–23.

[76] Rothenbacher, D., Kleiner, A., Koenig, W., Primatesta, P., Breitling, L. P., & Brenner, H. (2012). Relationship between inflammatory cytokines and uric acid levels with adverse cardiovascular outcomes in patients with stable coronary heart disease. PloS one, 7(9), e45907.

[77] Bogdanova A, Kaestner L. The Red Blood Cells on the Move!. Front Physiol. 2018;9:474. Published 2018 May 1. doi:10.3389/fphys.2018.00474

[78] Felker, G. Michael, et al. "Red Cell Distribution Width as a Novel Prognostic Marker in Heart FailureData From the CHARM Program and the Duke Databank." Journal of the American College of Cardiology 50.1 (2007): 40-47.

[79] Arbel, Yaron, et al. "Red blood cell distribution width and the risk of cardiovascular morbidity and all-cause mortality: a population-based study." European Heart Journal 34.suppl 1 (2013): P1549.

[80] Perlstein, Todd S., et al. "Red blood cell distribution width and mortality risk in a community-based prospective cohort." Archives of internal medicine 169.6 (2009): 588-594.

[81] Lewis, T., & Trempe, C. (2015). Chapter 6 – Science Behind Your Chronic Disease Temperature™. In Quarterback Your Own Health - How to Take and Lower Your Chronic Disease Temperature. Jefferson City, TN: Health Revival Partners. Available on Amazon.

[82] AREDS Research Group. (2004). Associations of mortality with ocular disorders and an intervention of high-dose antioxidants and zinc in the Age-Related Eye Disease Study: AREDS Report No. 13. Archives of ophthalmology, 122(5), 716.

[83] Vander, J. F. (2006). Progression of Age-Related Macular Degeneration: Prospective Assessment of C-Reactive Protein, Interleukin 6, and Other Cardiovascular Biomarkers Seddon JM, George S, Rosner B, et al (Massachusetts Eye and Ear Infirmary, Boston; Harvard Med School, Boston) Arch Ophthalmol 123: 774–782, 2005. Year Book of Ophthalmology, 2006, 114-115.

[84] Lewis, T., & Trempe, C. (2015). Chapter 4 – Your Eyes - Window to Your Health. In Quarterback Your Own Health - How to Take and Lower Your Chronic Disease Temperature. Jefferson City, TN: Health Revival Partners. Available on Amazon.

[85] Kljakovic, Marjan. "Patients and tests: A study into patient understanding of blood tests ordered by their doctor." Australian family physician 41, no. 4 (2012): 241.

Made in the USA
Columbia, SC
07 March 2021